IF YOU LIKE IT, DON'T EAT IT

By the same author

Cost-Effective Self-Sufficiency or The Middle-Class Peasant
  (with Eve McLaughlin)

Make Your Own Electricity

IF YOU LIKE IT, DON'T EAT IT

Dietary Fads and Fancies

Terence McLaughlin

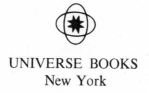

UNIVERSE BOOKS
New York

Published in the United States of America in 1979
by Universe Books
381 Park Avenue South, New York, N.Y. 10016

Library of Congress Catalog Card Number: 78–61206
ISBN 0–87663–332–7

Printed in Great Britain

Contents

1 Purists and Puritans

If you frequent health food stores, vegetarian restaurants, or any of the other haunts of those whose lives are dedicated to the pursuit of life, liberty and wholemeal bread, you will soon notice that most food reformers, like rugby players or theological students, tend to have a family resemblance.

It does not seem to matter much what their particular dietary theory may be—abstinence from meat or insistence on sea-salt, wholefoods or yang foods—they all carry around with them the air of being *committed*. You feel, as you look at the earnest bearded or scrubbed faces, that for these people life is too serious to be merely lived, and food too important to be casually eaten. Every activity has to be conducted carefully on the best theoretical principles, and those who take eating or living lightly must be Philistines or even enemies of the Truth. Strong passions are aroused by arguments about diet, and it is not uncommon to find people who have achieved oneness with the world by transcendental meditation in the morning wiping out all its good effects by getting uptight about potassium soup in the afternoon.

One of the reasons for this committed look, and the intensity of the passion, is that food reformers are usually also interested in a whole package of other causes, beside their chosen dietary system. In the 'twenties the popular package was typified by Bernard Shaw—vegetarianism went with Fabianism, Theosophy, penal reform, and the wearing of healthy Jaeger underwear. Now the trend is likely to be compounded of macrobiotic diet, Zen Buddhism, making electricity from windmills, educational reform, and wearing no panties, but the mood of high seriousness remains. Food reform is not just a way of preventing hunger, keeping healthy, or getting slim, and it is certainly a long way from the enjoyment of food for its own sake. Food has to be part of an attitude to life, a symptom of concern about the world and its deepest issues.

A revealing survey carried out by the UK Office of Health Economics in 1971 provides statistical evidence of this tendency to adopt a whole package of beliefs and mores as the natural accompaniment to a reformed diet. Vegetarians (meaning in this case ovolactovegetarians, who eat eggs and dairy products but no meat or fish) and vegans (those who abstain from all animals products) were questioned about their beliefs and opinions on a wide range of current problems, and their answers to the questionnaire were compared to those from a similarly-sized group of the general public. It was to be expected that such results would emerge as that 76 per cent of the vegans and 71 per cent of the vegetarians believed in the efficacy of herbal medicine, compared with only 32 per cent of the general population, but not so immediately obvious why 50 per cent of vegans and 45 per cent of vegetarians should support the Campaign for Nuclear Disarmament, while only 17 per cent of the public at large shared this view.

Over the survey as a whole, it turned out that vegetarians and vegans were mainly *for* herbalism, euthanasia, spiritualism and nuclear disarmament, and very much *against* vaccination, blood transfusion, immunization against disease, contraception, smoking, drinking, keeping pets, conducting animal experiments, and maintaining zoos. Oddly enough, fewer of the diet reformers subscribed to a belief in God than those in the control group, but this may have been because many of them are attracted to the Buddhist ethic which, in its uncorrupted form, does not involve a personal god.

Food reform is, therefore, a real moral issue for many of its devotees, and finds a place among other deeply-felt moral and social beliefs and opinions. I had an amusing example of this when I met a charming artist and his wife, both of fervent Radical Left views. We had been talking about the difficulty in knowing whether other people really care sincerely about the causes they publicly espouse, or if, as so often happens, they are merely jumping on the latest trendy band-waggon from the Sunday colour supplements. 'We had some friends who let us down like that,' said the wife, in tones of ultimate betrayal, 'We thought they were really sincere people, seriously concerned to improve the world. Then we discovered they didn't eat wholemeal bread.'

The books and magazines that cater for health-food enthusiasts also tend to offer a package of off-beat opinions on other topics. You constantly come across publishers' lists with books on diet juxtaposed with books on the occult, fringe medicine, radical politics, and other aspects of counter-culture. In a typical list you will see *The Vitamins Explained Simply* cheek-to-cheek with *Magic: Its Ritual Power and Purpose*: little radical magazines tell you how to make petrol bombs on one page, and where to buy free-range eggs on the next.

In the contents list of one of the magazines dealing with wholefoods and non-processed diet, I found the following grouping, with nothing to suggest that they were not all normal aspects of diet: 'Parsley—all-year-round vegetable', composting, vegetarian recipes, how to manage a small non-mechanized farm, keeping a goat . . . and then, at the end, 'Fairies, the hidden world of nature spirits'.

It was all very detailed, as well. Fairies are not, as I always imagined, confined to the bottom of the garden, along with the compost heaps and the things the dustmen will not take away. Fairies really prefer to hover round bulbs in bowls, occasionally waving their tentacles, which are pale grey. Poor little creatures. I imagine half the population, unaware of their status as nature spirits, has been spraying them with insecticide under the impression that they are woolly aphis.

Not all food reform literature goes to these lengths, of course, and you can find a great deal of sound sense in the books and magazines. However, there is this tendency to write on the assumption that diet enthusiasts are also automatically interested in astrology, fringe medicine, life in communes, alternative technology, are all opposed to factory farming and vivisection, and are all well on the way to being hypochondriacs. This is not a recent development: it is also present in vegetarian literature written before 1900, and in 1947 Bernard Shaw found it necessary to write a tart letter to the *British Vegetarian* about its tendency to lump together a rag-bag of radical views: 'What is needed is a Vegetarian journal that will ruthlessly separate fleshless diet from Humanitarianism, anti-War, Abolition of Capital Punishment, and all the usual sentimentalities that are associated with it. ONE THING AT A TIME.'

Unfortunately, Shaw was wrong in thinking that most of the readers of such magazines actually want one thing at a time—simple dietary information. The great majority of them seem to prefer their diets served up with a garnish of moral overtones, and side-dishes of all the miscellaneous reformist causes that happen to be fashionable. Those who adopt a new system of eating want it to be more than just a sensible or useful practice: they need to feel that it is ethically better, a new commandment engraved on stone tablets. The books and magazines, and many of their readers, exude an air of moral superiority more appropriate to a religion than to a mere matter of food.

This smugness seems to have been around for a long time. According to Greek myth, Hippolytus became a vegetarian in order to follow the cult of Orpheus, and obviously went around boring everyone to tears on the subject of righteous eating. When his father Theseus banished him on suspicion of adultery with Phaedra, Theseus seems to have got his own back for years of holier-than-thou attitudes—in Euripides' version of the story, he is made to say

> *Now* boast away, try to impress people with
> Your meatless meals . . .

The truth is that eating is something of a magical ceremony, even for materialistic Western man, and none of us can easily accept it as a mere mechanical or chemical process. We all tend, perhaps unconsciously, to read into our diet some kind of moral or spiritual value. How else but in a framework of magic could we reconcile ourselves to the fact that our continued existence depends on shovelling into ourselves bits of dead animals and things dug out of the ground?

All over the world, in less sophisticated societies, the magical nature of food is taken for granted. You are what you eat in very literal terms. The Wagogo men of south east Africa know for a fact that eating the heart of a lion will make them bold, while the heart of a hen will render them stupid and cowardly. Dyak warriors will not eat venison, in case they become as timid as the deer themselves. This is obviously not a normal taboo, or a hygienic rule based on the idea that deer are unclean, because the same people will willingly catch deer for women and old men to eat.

Perhaps the most striking example of this sympathetic magic in the selection of food is that recorded of Australian aborigines living in the bush. Despite a life so hard that insects, maggots, and similar creatures have to be pressed into service as food, the aborigines would not, even when nearly starving, eat tortoises, for fear of being slowed down in their hunting. On the other hand, the capture of a kangaroo evoked more enthusiasm than its weight in meat would justify, because such a swift animal would obviously improve the hunters' performance.

If you accept the tenets of sympathetic magic, and believe that the qualities of an animal pass into you along with its flesh, it becomes clear that cannibalism is not a sordid matter of necessity, but a compliment to the person who furnishes the meal. Most of the peoples who practised anthropophagy, except in periods of extreme famine, were hoping to absorb the bravery, wisdom, and other good qualities of their victims, and would not eat someone they despised. Much of this magical attitude has filtered through, in symbolic form, into modern religions—the rejection of pork by Jews and Moslems, or beef by Hindus, and even the symbolism of the Christian communion.

As Frazer, Lévi-Strauss, and many other anthropologists have shown, it is only a step from 'ordinary' cannibalism—eating a particular man whose bravery or other virtues are admired and coveted—to the ritual eating of certain animals and plants that are believed to embody the divine attributes of a god. As Frazer puts it (in his normal blunt anti-clerical way):

It is now easy to understand why a savage should desire to partake of the flesh of an animal or man whom he regards as divine. By eating the body of the god he shares in the god's attributes and powers. And when the god is a corn-god, the corn is his proper body; when he is a vine-god, the juice of the grape is his blood; and so by eating the bread and drinking the wine the worshipper partakes of the real body and blood of his god . . . Yet a time comes when reasonable men find it hard to understand how any one in his senses can suppose that by eating bread and drinking wine he consumes the body and blood of a deity.   (*The Golden Bough*, 1922 ed.)

However, reasonable men are not as numerous as Frazer imagined. So many of our beliefs about food turn out, when analysed, to be magical rather than logical, that we can hardly consider ourselves very much superior to Frazer's so-called savage. We may discount or explain away a literal interpretation of the communion, but how many times have you heard it said, for example, that 'good red meat' is essential for virility and energy? This has absolutely no basis in nutritional fact, and it is easily discovered that people can be healthy and virile on a diet with no meat at all, and certainly do not need the great bleeding chunks that figure so much in Western luxurious living. What the steak symbolizes is not a source of protein, but the potency and strength of the bull—a belief just about as rational as eating bread to absorb the spirit of the corn-god.

Similarly, most of the talk about 'natural' foods is a jumble of magic and pseudo-science. There are very real advantages in eating things that have not passed through the dark satanic mills of modern food-processing, but most of the claims made in the books and magazines directed at health-food enthusiasts seem to imply that corn-gods and vine-gods still exist, and can be confined to packets ready to serve up at mealtimes.

Every time we take up a new diet or food-fad, we are not just hoping to lose a few pounds in weight, or get a clearer skin, however much we may rationalize our motives on these lines. What we really expect, deep down, is that the new diet will bring about a new life, miraculously absorbed through some exotic food, or earned by noble abstinence from the things we really enjoy eating but feel are 'bad for us'. A convincing dietary system has to appeal, not primarily to our reasoning faculties, but to the magical and primitive sides of our nature. If you want to think up a new dietary system (and there are many less profitable occupations), throw your textbooks on nutrition out of the window. Concentrate on two basic elements—ritual and sacrifice.

The ritual can be something quite simple—Horace Fletcher made himself a household name merely by recommending people to chew every mouthful until it was completely pulped and depressingly tasteless. It may be a system that needs tables and charts, like the macrobiotic diet with its yin foods and yang foods, that sends its Western disciples scouring the shops for expensively-imported Japanese food, while ignoring home-grown products of almost exactly equal food value. Magic ingredients are always popular—cider vinegar, blackstrap molasses, yoghurt, honey, comfrey, wheatgerm, bran—or you can set up for yourself a daily routine in which certain foods or supplements have to be taken at set hours, like the observances in a monastery. When a popular romantic novelist describes her daily ritual of taking ninety vitamin or mineral pills, plus a 'brain pill', two ginseng tablets, and a cup of ginseng tea, one is reminded less of dietary matters than of a devout *religieuse* reciting Hail Marys.

The sacrifice aspect of diet is perhaps even more important than the ritual. Quite the best way to make a name in the diet and health press is to come out with a diatribe against some particular food, the more popular the better. Sugar, meat, tea, coffee, bread, milk and fried foods of all kinds have been condemned in one system or another, and if you believed all the diet writers over, say, the last hundred years, you would probably decide that it was simpler not to eat at all.

The language used to describe the offending foods is often religious in its intensity—you are reminded of John Knox denouncing idolatry, or General Booth proscribing alcohol. There are no half-tones or doubts—everything is black and white. People, according to the diet reformers, do not just drink tea or coffee, or eat white sugar or white bread. They are 'tea-addicts', 'coffee-addicts', 'self–poisoners with sugar', and so on. White bread is not considered as something rather inferior to wholemeal bread, but completely, ineluctably bad. 'Bread is the staff of death rather than life,' said Emmet Densmore in 1890, and the phrase has been copied enthusiastically by succeeding generations of diet writers.

A fine example of this Old Testament denunciatory style is the book *Superior Nutrition* by Herbert M. Shelton (published by Dr Shelton's Health School, Texas, 1951). Dr Shelton is a pioneer of the 'Natural Hygiene' diet (or rather, non-diet, because his main therapeutic technique appears to be prolonged fasting). Witness Dr Shelton on the subject of other dietitians' methods, and note the strong resemblance to Jeremiah denouncing the children of Israel: 'Our people are drunk on food excess and the dietitians encourage them to eat more. They provide trick diets of one kind or another, designed to give them variations in their gluttony, but they never admonish the people to discontinue their gluttony . . .'

As bad as too much food, in Dr Shelton's eyes, is the sinful attempt to bring variety into meals: '. . . this is especially true of those on the conventional diet of *stimulating* foods. They establish a nervous 'craving' for *stimulation* which is referred to the stomach for satisfaction and is in every way like the 'craving' of the drunkard for his alcohol or of the morphine addict for his morphine.'

It seems, in fact, as if sacrifice is something that strongly attracts food reformers—or perhaps that food reform attracts those who already have an ascetic attitude towards life. At every period, writers who set themselves up to inculcate a 'better' system of diet seem also anxious to impose other penances on their disciples, and even to remove any element of pleasure from the act of eating itself: 'If a man will take his pleasure from eating and drinking, he will have none in life' as J. P. Sandlands, an early nature-cure enthusiast put it in his book *Health—A Royal Road to It* (1909), a text unusually thorough even for its time in its depressing emphasis on the duty to make eating as dull as possible.

Bronson Alcott, a friend of Emerson and father of Louisa May Alcott the writer, had the same austere approach to food: 'As to my accepted bill of fare, I may add, moreover, that fruits rank first and foremost in the pyramid; bread, properly, next; and vegetables lowest. Sobriety in all pleasures is the open way to the highest and purest satisfactions; the deepest, holiest this life can give.'

Small wonder that Carlyle described Alcott as 'a venerable Don Quixote, all bent on saving the world by a return to acorns and the golden age'. For those nearer home, like his wife Abigail May and their four daughters, sobriety in all pleasures seems to have palled. In later life Louisa May defined a philosopher as 'a man up in a balloon, with his family and friends holding the ropes which confine him to earth and trying to haul him down,' but there must have been days when the Alcott family could cheerfully have let go the ropes and seen their sober father disappear for ever.

Early in the twentieth century, when temperance and prohibition were far more fashionable platforms than they are now, they were often considered as the natural concomitant of vegetarianism and similar dietary systems. For example, the Rev J. C. Street addressed the Vegetarian Society of Manchester on *The Humane Principle* in 1903, and his first sentence ran 'Being a life-long abstainer from intoxicants, vegetarianism has always had some attraction for me'. This approach seems to have caused no sense of incongruity among his audience. Indeed, the hyper-ascetic approach to food and drink was very popular among food reformers, and this was the aspect that most impressed itself on the public at large and the press, when they thought about diet reform at all. The stock cartoon vegetarian was a wild-haired figure in sandals and rough tweeds, with a sour expression and a general attitude of cold negation—a sort of homespun Mrs Grundy.

G. K. Chesterton, a lover of beer and good food, and, to be fair, logic, lampooned the movement in many of his books and essays, and in *The Flying Inn* drew a characteristically fantastic satirical picture of an England in which vegetarianism and prohibition have been imposed together by a group of ascetic

legislators. Here is Captain Dalroy, the chief rebel against the
new regime, pointing out how illogical the amalgamation of the
two systems is in fact:

> And, now I come to think of it, if I'm to be a vegetarian,
> why shouldn't I drink? Why shouldn't I have a purely
> vegetarian drink? Why shouldn't I take vegetables in their
> highest form, so to speak? The modest vegetarians ought
> obviously to stick to wine or beer, plain vegetarian drinks,
> instead of filling their goblets with the blood of bulls and
> elephants, as all conventional meat-eaters do, I suppose.

This gives an excuse for the well-known song with verses such as

> You will find me drinking rum,
> Like a sailor in a slum,
> You will find me drinking beer like a Bavarian;
> You will find me drinking gin
> In the lowest kind of inn,
> Because I am a rigid Vegetarian.

But despite Chesterton's noisy fun about the coalition between
vegetarianism and other kinds of abstinence, they tended to
grow even closer together. Diet reform became even more
firmly wedded to a general movement towards asceticism. The
young lawyer Mohandas Gandhi, long before his great nation-
alist work for India, joined with the dietitian Dr Josiah Oldfield
to start a London Vegetarian Club, as a counterpart to the
already flourishing Vegetarian Society in Manchester, and both
of them obviously regarded diet as one aspect of a complete
philosophy of moderation and austerity. Gandhi later set out
his theories of vegetarianism as the proper way to a spirit of
non-violence and the subjugation of 'animal instincts' of all
kinds, particularly sexual instincts:

> Abstemiousness from intoxicating drinks and drugs, and
> from all kinds of foods, especially meat, is undoubtedly a
> great aid to the evolution of the spirit . . .
> Experience teaches that animal food is unsuited to those
> who would curb their passions.

Dr Oldfield went even further, and in *Eat and Be Happy* (1929) not only proscribes alcohol, but even beans, on the basis that these may have unduly exciting effects:

A large use of legumens is to be avoided—beans, peas, lentils etc., are valuable foods, but in connexion with their high protein contents there is an obscure element which acts as an excitant upon the procreative cells.

The observation of centuries has concentrated its experience into an apothegm when it sums up a youth at the exploding point of self-control as being 'full of beans'.

As we shall see in the next chapter, Pythagoras had similar views about beans and their effects on the sexual impulses: for Dr Oldfield any suggestion of such unseemliness was enough to ensure the banishment of the bean from his diet—he was in fact strongly antagonistic to sex in any form except for the express purpose of continuing the human race. Tolstoy had similar views, and in *The First Step* equated meat-eating with promiscuous sex: '[Meat] is quite unnecessary, and only serves to develop animal feelings, to excite desire, to promote fornication and drunkenness'.

Emmet Densmore, writing his book *How Nature Cures—The Natural Food of Man* in 1892, actually broke into a cry from the heart that would have delighted both Tolstoy and Dr Oldfield: 'If mankind could in a day be persuaded to refrain from indulgence in the sexual relation except for the purposes of procreation, an amazing improvement, in greater freedom from nervous diseases and all diseased conditions . . . would be at once manifest.' This seems to have very little to do with diet and nature-cure, but a great deal to do with Dr Densmore's own reasons for recommending an ascetic approach to food.

Even in 1489, the the *Governayle of Helthe* (see pages 26–8), it seems to have been impossible to get away from the notion that diet reform was identified with sexual abstinence (restraint from alcohol was perhaps unthinkable at the time, if only because of the very doubtful water supplies in most places). At the end of the treatise the author breaks into doggerel verse, of which the first lines run

> For helth of body, covere for cold thy hede
> Ete no rawe mete, take good hede hereto,
> Drynke holsom wyne. Fede the on lyght brede
> Wyth an appetyte ryse from thy mete also,
> *Wyth wymmen fleshely have not adoo*   (my italics)

In the pages that follow many dietary systems appear, some simple, others complicated, some sensible, others perverse to the point of being dangerous. But in all of them the two magic elements appear in some degree—*ritual*, the belief that good can only come from the system if certain prescribed foods or actions are used, and *sacrifice*, the belief that the only true way to salvation is to give up some or all of the pleasures of life, and particularly any form of food or drink that is popularly enjoyed.

The history of diet reveals a constant struggle between the hedonists and the ascetics: the hedonists would no doubt side with the Spanish king described in this seventeenth-century account 'Alphonsus, King of Aragon, having heard by what maner of diet one had atteined to 90 yeeres of age, replied, that hee had rather die within ten yeeres then live an hundred yeeres by means of so strict a diet . . .'

The ascetics, on the other hand, would say, with Goethe

> Entbehren sollst du, sollst entbehren!
> Das ist der ewige Gesang.   (*Faust*, I)
> (You must abstain, you must abstain,
> That is the eternal song.)

And, despite the temptation, we must all abstain from drawing too obvious a conclusion from the fact that the hedonist was called Alfonso the Wise, while the spokesman for the ascetics was Mephistopheles.

2 Classical Restraint

No matter how wretched the lives of people may be, there are always those reformers who are ready to tell them that further austerity is the only way to salvation; no matter how limited their diet, there are always some foods which are denounced as unfit for use, for magical, religious, or hygienic reasons. Tribes who eke out a miserable existence on worms, grubs and centipedes may still refuse to eat tortoise or some other taboo animal, and in modern India, with the greater part of the population near starvation most of the time, there is no lack of teachers to inform the people that their troubles arise from over-indulgence.

It seems that this has always been so, even among the earliest creatures we can confidently call men. While man was showing his superior survival power over the other primates by extending the repertoire of foods he would try eating, he was also developing the mental concept of taboo, which prevented him from making use of some quite suitable sources of food for totally irrational motives.

These taboos did not grow up as a result of unpleasant experiences with poisonous plants or animals—indeed, one of the remarkable things about early man was the speed with which he developed quite complicated processes to render such materials fit to eat. The manioc tuber, for example, is a rich source of starch, but unsuitable for normal use because of the hydrogen cyanide (prussic acid) it contains. This poison can be removed by soaking the sliced or chopped roots in water and then squeezing out and disposing of the juice: this process seems to have been known to some peoples in Mesolithic periods, or at least 4000 BC. Taboo is a far more complicated psychological and sociological process than the simple avoidance of overtly harmful things, and anthropologists are still arguing about the nature of it in their usual quarrelsome way. However, the results of it are clear—certain foods became, in every real sense, uneatable to certain tribes, despite the fact that the foods might have made the difference between death and life in simple nutritional terms.

Religion, and the psychological bias towards austerity that has already been considered in the previous chapter, have often had a similar effect of inducing people to give up some part of even the simplest diet in the hopes of spiritual benefit.

In ancient Greece, for example, the average family lived on a very plain and sparing diet. Even in metropolitan Athens the citizens, although they might be blessed with the words of Sophocles, Euripides, or Alcaeus, and the music of Terpander, tended to live on a diet of wheat or barley bread and thick soups or stews made of lentils, peas, beans, and similar pulses, enlivened by the occasional onion, clove of garlic, or radish. According to Pliny, poor people, with no means of cooking for themselves, often had just bread, olive oil, and an occasional helping of hot thick soup or pudding made from chick-peas or lupin seeds and sold in the streets.

Even among the richer people, meat was a rare dish, although they had eggs and fish. Most families only tasted meat when there was a festival for a god, or a wedding or some similar family celebration, and then quite often a group of families would form a club (*eranos*=a contribution) to buy a lamb or sheep to be slaughtered and cooked in the open. There was a special and respected profession of *mageiros*, both butcher and cook, who would take charge of the whole operation, as very few people knew how to cook meat, it being eaten so seldom.

Greek food was essentially simple even for the rich, and there were none of the elaborate concocted dishes which are familiar in later Roman descriptions of meals. The flavourings and dressings were limited to onions, garlic, coriander, sesame and vinegar, and about the most elaborate dish was fish served on a plate with a depression for a sauce in the middle. In the country game such as hares, deer, and wild boars gave occasional variety, but this was strictly a rich man's meat: Xenophon and Menander in their writing on sport make it clear that only the wealthy could afford to hunt.

With a diet of such simplicity, it is difficult to see at first how any more restricted one was possible, but the Greeks had in fact a long tradition of vegetarianism for religious reasons. The cult of Orpheus required that animals should not be killed, even for sacrifice to the gods, and the teachings of Pythagoras (c 586–506 BC) laid even greater emphasis on the 'blood-brotherhood' between men and animals.

Pythagoras was strongly influenced by the Orphic cults, and by the eastern doctrine of the 'wheel of life' and reincarnation which forms such an important part of Buddhist and Hindu theology. As the quality of every person's life (the *karma*, as it is now called) decided whether the next incarnation would be higher or lower in enlightenment, a wicked or unfortunate life might result in the person returning as an animal—'the soul of our grandma might haply inhabit a bird', as Shakespeare says facetiously in *Twelfth Night*. Hence it was important not to kill any living thing for food or sacrifice. He was also a believer in the power of asceticism to set the soul free from the wheel of life and the constant round of new existences, and made his disciples not only refrain from meat and milk, but also from such common Greek fare as beans. (This may have been from the belief, already described, that beans caused sexual desires, and also, in an allegorical sense, a direction that his followers should not meddle with politics, as beans were used for casting votes in ancient Greek society.)

His white-clad followers soon became known all over Greece because of their unthinking allegiance to the Master and their abstinent habits, rather as the acolytes of the Hare Krishna movement are noticed today, and for the same reasons. At one time there were reputed to be around 2,600 Pythagorean disciples in one college. Plato's *Phaedo* describes the general theology on right living and thinking as expressed by the Pythagoreans, and Ovid, writing about their attitude to diet in the *Metamorphoses*, book 15, looks back over the intervening

500 years and casts a nostalgic glow over the character of Pythagoras:

> There was a man in the town, Pythagoras, who was born in Samos, but fled the island and its tyrant, and because of his hatred of tyranny went into exile . . . He was the first to forbid the serving of animal food at meals, and first to preach as follows—wise words, but with little effect on his audience—'Fellow men, do not pollute your bodies with such impious food. You have the fruits of the earth, you have apples bending down the branches with their weight, and grapes ripening on the vines. You have delicious herbs and vegetables which can be cooked and softened over the fire, and you are not short of milk, or honey fragrant with the scent of thyme. The earth is generous with her wealth, and supplies you with kindly sustenance without any need for bloodshed or killing . . . How criminal it is to cram flesh into our own flesh, for one greedy body to grow fat at the expense of another, to go on living only by the destruction of other lives!'

Lucian of Samosata, the Swift of his age, and much harder-edged than the romantic Ovid, found Pythagoras and his doctrines a subject for satire in *The Sale of Lives*: here is the philosopher justifying his theories on diet:

> Pythagoras: I am a vegetarian, and I do not eat beans either.
>
> Customer: Why not? Do they make you ill?
>
> Pythagoras: No, but the bean is holy. It helps reproduction. If you peel a bean when it is sprouting you will see that it is exactly like the male sexual organs. If you cook it and expose it to the moon for the exact number of nights it will turn to blood. Besides, beans are used in Athens to vote at elections . . .

(The notion that beans turn to blood is found in a great deal of folklore. Brigid Brophy and others have pointed out that this could be due to the fact that when most varieties of bean are boiled, the water turns dark red.)

By the time Ovid and Lucian wrote about the founder of vegetarianism, both his diet and his ideas of moderation in food must have seemed very strange and old-fashioned. The Roman Empire was a place for gluttons, and the Greeks who were influenced by their Roman masters became almost as gross in their tastes. In Rome itself the mark of a rich man was the elaboration and expense of his dinner table: Apicius, for example, who is said to have spent a hundred million sesterces on food, and committed suicide when he found that he had only ten million left. Apicius is credited with what are probably the first two cookery books, one on main dishes and the other on sauces (although the books actually published under his name are probably later compilations). From these books we can learn the haute cuisine of Rome—seventeen ways to cook a sucking pig, stuffed marrows, asparagus purée served with eggs, snails force-fed on milk until they are so fat that they cannot get back in their shells (*ut non possint se retrahere*) and so on.

This last technique is typical of the sophistication of imperial Roman food production: delicacies were used in such profusion that they had to be 'factory farmed'. For instance, large perforated jars were used to maintain intensive breeding of 'battery' dormice for the table: dormice in honey was a popular dish, but Apicius describes a more elaborate preparation in which the dormouse is cleaned and then stuffed with a mixture of minced pork and dormouse meat, pepper, pine kernels, asafoetida, and fish sauce (*liquamen*). To give them distinctive flavours, the dormice could be fed on various fodder: acorns produced a cheap, plain dormouse, but chestnuts or walnuts gave a more expensive and tasty animal.

For a great banquet, no expense was spared. Petronius' 'Trimalchio's Feast' episode in the *Satyricon* gives a good idea of a banquet in a household where money is abundant and good taste almost entirely absent. One of the dishes is the so-called Trojan Pig. Host Trimalchio sends for a pig to be brought in from the kitchen, and when it arrives the host and the cook keep up the pretence that the kitchen staff have forgotten to gut the pig before cooking it:

'Well,' said Trimalchio, 'As you forgot to do it before, gut the pig in front of us.'

The cook took up his knife and with nervous hands slit the pig open right and left. Suddenly the slits widened, and out came a collection of sausages and black puddings . . .

Fish, though common enough in the rest of Italy, was a luxury in the city of Rome itself, so characteristically the rich diners demanded fish which sometimes cost ridiculous prices: one host paid seven or eight thousand sesterces for a single red mullet, and Cato says that even in the second century BC a fish could cost more than a cow.

Every now and then legislation was passed in a vain attempt to cut down the extravagance on food. Julius Caesar, for instance, passed a law in 46 BC which forbade the sale of some of the more exotic foods, and introduced a limit to the amount a household could spend on meat. Such laws had very little result: the counter to this particular one was to make up a number of very elaborate dishes based only on vegetables, which were not restricted. Cicero recorded going to one such 'vegetarian' dinner and eating so much that he was very ill the next day. In practice the various sumptuary laws were ignored, and only very spasmodic attempts were made to enforce them.

Even outside the class of very rich epicures, with their conspicuous consumption of rare foods brought from all over the Empire, a good Roman dinner in early imperial times was quite a luxurious affair. The first course was usually hors d'oeuvres (*gustatio*)—olives, sliced eggs, shellfish and *beche de mer*, snails, sausages and meat puddings, with lettuce, leeks, mint and other herbs for flavouring. The Romans ate small onions, but apparently garlic was not much liked—it was more characteristic of Greek cookery.

The main course (*cena*) consisted of a number of made-up dishes brought round in rotation, usually three 'waves' of service, for the guests to choose from. Game birds were popular —pheasant and wild goose—hare, wild boar (most hosts would serve a leg of boar, the whole animal was a dish indulged in only by the very rich), ham, stuffed lamb, and fish. Lamprey and turbot were quite commonly served, though more expensive than a meat dish. Beef was not common on good tables, mainly because not many animals were bred for meat; the cattle used near Rome were mostly draught animals, which would have been very tough, and milch-cows, too valuable to kill and eat. However, pork was popular, as was dog—dogs were fattened especially for the table and prepared rather as if they were large hares.

Finally a dessert (*bellaria*) would be served: apples, grapes, nuts, figs, and pears. Pears were brought all the way from Syria, wrapped in straw to preserve them.

While among the regular gluttons the *vomitorium* was occasionally used to relieve an overloaded stomach so that its owner could go on eating, this was probably not such a common custom as has been supposed. Obviously some guests would make themselves sick by drinking too much wine, as still happens sometimes today. Seneca, like most satirists, tended to take the worst view of his contemporaries: 'People eat to vomit, and vomit to eat; their food is brought from every corner of the world, and then they do not even bother to digest it.'

However, even if this criticism was over-sour, there is no doubt that the Romans were unrefined eaters. They had the custom, which remained in Europe generally for some centuries after, of throwing left-overs on to the floor—the legs and shells of lobsters, shells from snails, apple cores, bits of gristle and so on—so that servants or slaves were constantly sweeping up during a big dinner. The visual effect was so fascinating that an artist called Sosus became very fashionable by making mosaic pavements with the debris already depicted (*asarotos oikos*= the unswept pavement), of which several still exist in museums.

The Romans were also keenly interested in food, and it was not unusual for the guests to gather in the kitchen to see some special dish being prepared. The exchange of recipes, and gossip about the eccentricities of cooks, were common topics for men's conversation at dinner, and Varro, the satirist, remarked that if only the Romans would spend on philosophy a tenth of the time they spent on talking about the baking of bread, they would be much better morally and intellectually.

Naturally enough, the serious-minded Romans saw in all

this luxury and frivolity the seeds of decline. Many writers contrasted the vast expense of a metropolitan dinner with the simple life of the peasant, who managed quite well on a diet of millet soup, coarse bread, and a few turnips, olives, beans, figs, and perhaps some cheese. Seneca the Younger actually lived a vegetarian life for some years, and wrote about it to Lucilius: 'I . . . began to abstain from animal food, and by the end of one year I found this habit as pleasant as it was easy.'

He gave up the diet, not from any distaste for it, but because in the reign of Tiberius vegetarianism was associated with religious cults such as the worship of Isis. As so often, religion became mixed with politics, and Tiberius saw the cults as a threat to the state. So, as Seneca says: ' . . . abstinence from certain kinds of animal food was set down as a proof of interest in the strange religion. At the request of my father, who was not afraid of prosecution but detested philosophical arguments, I returned to my previous diet.'

Even so, Seneca maintained a very sparing regime for the rest of his life, and lived mainly on vegetables plainly cooked, with very little meat. This made him even more critical of the excesses that he occasionally saw going on round him. As he was so well known for austerity, a number of legends about him began to gather—Thomas Muffet related a curious anecdote in *Healths Improvement* (1655): 'It is recorded by *St Jerom* in his Epistles, that *Seneca* upon a foolish conceit abstained so long from flesh, and fed only upon fruit and fish . . . that when upon *Neroes* commandment he was to bleed to death, there did not spring from him a drop of blood.'

The Simple Life had other proponents: Horace constantly drew contrasts between the unhealthy hurry and intrigue of the city and the peaceful contemplation of the country, and is careful to make it clear that country life means country food:

> If, my Torquatus, you will kindly deign
> To lie on couches roughly made and plain,
> And sup on herbs alone, though richly dressed,
> I shall be pleased to see you as my guest . . .

> (*Letters*, I, 5)

However, one senses that Horace's attitude to the simple life was about as sincere as that of Pope. His existence on his little farm in the Sabine hills was very much that of a comfortable country gentleman, and he kept extremely close touch with the fashions and follies of the city, while satirizing them.

One interesting aspect of the imperial Roman diet is that there does not seem to have been any equivalent of the modern fallacious belief that athletes need large quantities of meat to keep them fit and strong. The gladiators were fed generously while in their barracks, and in fact it was a recognized thing that anyone in Rome who was actually starving could always sign on as a gladiator, thus ensuring a well-fed life, if a short one, but the food itself was coarse and simple, mostly barley and beans with the very occasional piece of pork.

Again, in contrast to the later European belief that invalids must somehow have meat forced down them if they are to recover, the diet for Roman patients was kept sensibly light, with a good deal of fruit and vegetables—fresh peas, lentils and figs were particularly recommended, with soft-boiled eggs, shellfish, and a little chicken. Galen and Celsus, the two greatest medical authorities of the Roman Empire, spent a great deal of space in their textbooks on the diet for various types of disease, and in general their recommendations are extremely sensible. In some cases they even achieved genuine cures by diet, one of the most remarkable treatments being the cure of night-blindness and sore eyes by administration of ox liver in honey (a treatment which actually dated back to Hippocrates of Cos, around 400 BC). The night-blindness, now called *nyctalopia*, and sore eyes (*xerophthalmia*), are both symptoms of vitamin A deficiency: the Roman diet would have been rather short of the vitamin except among those who ate eggs regularly—carrots, the best vegetable source, were known, but were probably very small and tough compared with the modern root, and used only as a garnish for other food. Liver, however, contains a great deal of the vitamin, and even a small amount would ensure an apparently miraculous cure of the eye troubles.

Unfortunately, not all of the theories of Galen, in particular, were as sound. Like many doctors in modern times, Galen had delusions of omniscience, and had also inherited from the Greek Peripatetic philosophers the habit of spinning out his theories in a fine chain of logical premises until they had lost all touch with reality. While Celsus was keeping hospital patients happy and healthy with a fruit diet, Galen's theories led him to the view that fruit was unhealthy and caused fevers. This was probably because fruit was usually available during the heat of the summer and autumn, when fevers were also most common because of the proliferation of bacteria, and also because the diarrhoeas occasionally caused by fruit seemed to be linked to the symptoms of fevers such as dysentery. Whatever the reasons, Galen put the stamp of his authority on the condemnation of fruit, and the sheer volume of his writing (500 treatises) ensured that his authority was not questioned for many centuries to come. Like the spirit of Aristotle in philosophy, the spirit of Galen can be sensed brooding over the whole history of diet and medicine until about the seventeenth century, and some of his theories (not always the correct ones) may be seen lurking in the background of books on diet even today.

3 Feast Days and Fast Days

Roman society had its share of criticism from within, from satirists like Horace or misanthropists like Seneca, but it was also watched over with a far from friendly eye by the early Christians. As, most of the time, Imperial Rome was the enemy, there was a tendency for everything Roman to be regarded as unchristian. Sometimes this led to absurd and unpleasant consequences, as when St Benedict, who regarded the public baths at Rome as a hotbed of vice, declared that bathing in general was sinful—'to those that are well, and especially to the young, bathing shall seldom be permitted'—and several saints were canonized for no better reason than that they had lived a life so austere that water had never touched them after their baptism.

The rules of St Benedict also restricted diet, and the order of monks which he founded were supposed to abstain from all flesh meat, although they were allowed fish and eggs. This was not such a stringent austerity as it might seem now: Benedict came from Nursia, a small village near Spoleto, c AD 480, and while he himself came from a family rich enough to send him to Rome to school, the people round him must have been used to a largely meatless diet.

However, there is much evidence that Benedict's rules for monastic life were largely ignored. An account by Giraldus Cambrensis of a visit to Canterbury in about 1170 shows that life in a large monastery could be extremely luxurious, and there were even ways of getting over the problems of the prohibition on speaking at meals:

As he sat there at the high table with the Prior and the seniors, he noted two things, the multitude of dishes and the excessive superfluity of signs which the monks made to one another. For there was the Prior giving so many dishes to the serving monks, and they in their turn bearing these as gifts to the lower tables; and there were those, to whom these gifts were brought, offering their thanks, and all of them gesticulating with fingers, hands, and arms, and whistling to one another in lieu of speaking, all extravagating in a manner more free and frivolous than was seemly . . .

. . . sixteen very costly dishes or even more were placed upon the table in order, or rather contrary to all order. Finally vegetables were brought to every table, but were not much eaten. For you might see so many kinds of fish, roast and boiled, stuffed and fried, so many dishes contrived with eggs and pepper by dexterous cooks, so many sauces and condiments, made up with equal skill to tickle gluttony and awaken appetite. Moreover there were wines, metheglin, claret, must, mead and mulberry juice, drinks so choice that beer, which is at its best in England and particularly in Kent, was despised like the vegetables.

The clergy in general expected to live well, and had food which was not only superior in quantity but in quality to that of their parishioners. This gave rise to a set of class-prejudices about food that are illustrated amusingly by a story in *Moralitates* by Thomas Waleys (*c* 1330): a bishop wanted a new fishpond dug on his land, and recruited local labour from the village. Being a kindly man, and also wanting his pond dug quickly, he arranged to send out bread from his own household, good wheaten bread which he hoped would please the workmen. Within a few days he found the work proceeding very slowly, and when he enquired the reason, was told that the men were hungry and weak. Angry with his steward, the bishop insisted that he had ordered bread to be issued. 'That is not bread for the likes of us,' said the peasants, 'We don't call that real bread. Give us good bean-bread and we shall be able to work.'

For the majority of the population of medieval Europe, food

was in chronically short supply, and it seems strange that diet
fads could arise under the circumstances—however, the story
above shows how little encouragement people need to become
choosy about their diet. An extremely popular treatise on food
in early medieval times was the *Regimen Sanitatis Salerni*,
written some time in the twelfth century and summing up
several centuries of medical teaching at Salerno, the centre of
European medical skill for about 1,300 years. The treatise was
said to have been compiled for Robert of Normandy, eldest
son of William the Conquerer, but it is probably earlier writings
which were hastily recopied and dedicated to Robert when he
passed through Salerno on his way to the first Crusade. Many
copies of this work circulated in the monasteries during the
fourteenth and fifteenth centuries, and the treatise was still
very popular in Jacobean times, when Sir John Harington,
Queen Elizabeth's godson, translated it into English as *The
Englishman's Doctor, or The School of Salernum* (1608).
Harington's versified edition gives a good idea of the doctrines
of the Regimen in quite amusing couplets: on milk, for instance

> In great consumptions learn'd Physicians thinke,
> 'Tis good a *Goat* or *Camels* milke to drinke,
> *Cowes-milke* and *Sheepes* doe well, but yet an *Asses*
> Is best of all, and all the other passes.

Johannes de Mirfeld of St Bartholomew's, Smithfield, had
much the same to say in the fourteenth century, and was
possibly also copying his ideas from the *Regimen*:

> Milk is of the greatest possible value [for consumptives],
> especially human milk: asses milk comes next in value, and
> then that of goats. The milk ought if possible to be taken
> direct from the udder, but if this is out of the question the
> animal should be milked into a salver which is held over
> another salver full of hot water, and the milk given to the
> patient immediately, for it quickly goes bad. . .

Cheese, a great source of protein for working men, was considered a 'hot and dry' food, and not recommended for invalids:

For healthie men new *Cheese* be wholesome food,
But for the weake and sickly 'tis not good,
Cheese is an heavie meate, both grosse and cold
And breedeth Costivenesse both new and old . . .

(Harington)

Harington seems a little confused here, as a little later in the verse he says that cheese 'helps a stomach cold to warm', which would agree with the account of it in the *Regimen*. New cheese at the time would have been a kind of soft cream or cottage cheese, often called *green cheese* because of its youth, not its colour, and *spermyse*, cottage cheese flavoured with herbs. Hard cheese was of the Cheddar type, rennet cheese hardened by pressure and allowed to mature.

Another very popular treatise was the *Governayle of Helthe* (1489), an anonymous work in English originally printed by Caxton. This is a complete guide to healthy living—diet, exercise, and even what one might call 'positive thinking'—which rather surprisingly breaks into doggerel verse near the end, presumably to provide a summary of the main points in a memorable form. Like most of the medical literature of the time, it leans heavily on Galen, and much of the detailed advice is rather nonsensical, depending as it does on Galen's chop-logic reasoning rather than observation, but the general rules of health which are stated are quite sound—moderation in eating and drinking, taking enough exercise, not eating when depressed or angry, and so on. The writer gives eight golden rules—seven very general and the eighth curiously specialized:

. . . viii thynges at the leste ben nedefull in holsome governayle, of which the fyrste is a dyscrete choys of thos thynges that shall be eten or dronken; the seconde is wylfull bodyli exercice to fore mete, and that tyl the swetyng begynne . . .; the thirde is well profytable and wel nedeful that all that shall be etyn be well and smale chewed; the fourth is that thou ete while thou has talent [appetite] to ete; the *v* is that thou slepe on morow [morning] tyl thou wake be thyne owne wytt. For as Aristotle sayth, not only in metys and drynkys be we noryshed and fostred, but also in slepe. The *vi* is that

thou take no mete and drynk in sorow ne in care but in Joye
as moche as thou maye; the *vii* is that thou have ne holde nor
colde in wynter ne in somer after bloodletynge; the *viii* is
that thou use Saffron in thy mete, for it quycneth kyndely
hete and comforteth thy dygestyon & taryeth thyne elde or
age and bryngeth in gladnes, and letteth thyne humors from
rotynge and driynge.

The last encomium on saffron sounds almost like an advertising claim for a new wonder drug: it has always been considered a valuable flavouring, and was much in demand for
addition to food in the sixteenth century. However, Culpeper,
while saying it is 'endowed with great virtues', warns his readers
not to take too much, 'for when the dose is too large, it
produces a heaviness of the head and sleepiness; some have
fallen into an immoderate convulsive laughter, which ended in
death.'

The *Governayle of Helthe* classified foods according to the
Doctrine of Humours, a system first introduced by Hippocrates
and vastly elaborated by Galen, which dominated medieval
medical and psychological thinking. Individuals were divided
into four different types, sanguine, phlegmatic, choleric or
melancholic, and their type was a measure both of their
appearance and their personality. For example, sanguine people
were ruddy-faced, fleshy, inclined to sleep long, optimistic in
temperament and unsubtle in thought: 'The veins of their eyes
be red, as well as their faces. They are much inclined to laughter,
witty and merry, conceited in discourse, pleasant, if they be
not far gone, much given to music, dancing, and to be in
women's company.' (Burton, *The Anatomy of Melancholy*).
Phlegmatic people, on the other hand are 'dull, slow, cold,
blockish, ass-like . . . they delight in waters, ponds, pools,
rivers, fishing, fowling, etc'. (Burton).

These types were supposed to arise from a certain mixing of
qualities, hot, cold, moist and dry, which led to the dominant
humour, blood, phlegm, yellow or green bile, and black bile, so
that the doctor could take one look at his patient and classify
him from the following table:

Type	Qualities	Humour
Sanguine	Hot and moist	Blood
Phlegmatic	Cold and moist	Phlegm
Choleric	Hot and dry	Yellow or green bile
Melancholic	Cold and dry	Black bile

Foods were also supposed to have the *qualities* of heat, cold, moistness or dryness, and the art of diet was to give each person foods which would counteract any excess of the qualities in his make-up. Lettuce, for example, was considered cold and moist (reasonably enough) and therefore ideal food for choleric young men (hot and dry) but not for phlegmatic old men (also cold and moist) (see also pp 125–6). Sanguine or choleric people were not recommended to eat much of 'hot' foods: in the *Governayle* these are represented by 'peper, garlek, oynyons, cresses, sauge, myntes, persile and suche other,' while cold foods were 'letuse, pursilan, gourdes and suche other'.

Intricate reasoning was used to find a suitable classification of qualities for every article of food, or herb used in medicine, and to give even greater scope for ingenious rationalizations, a system of *degrees* was added to the qualities: cabbage, for example, was considered hot in the first degree but dry only in the second degree, so that while it was completely unsuitable for those of a choleric humour, and rather unsuitable for those of a sanguine humour, it was probably just about acceptable for those who were melancholic, because the 'dryness' was not excessive. With such a system, based almost entirely on complicated verbal games and very little on practical experience, the most important attribute for a doctor was an ability to read the authorities, such as Galen. Andrew Boorde, in his *Breviarie of Health* (1552) outlines the necessary learning for a doctor of his time: a physician must have 'Grammer to understand what he doth read in Latin . . . but above all things next to Grammer, a Physitian must have surely his Astronimy, to know, how, when and at what time everye medicine ought to be ministred'.

While there were some successes from the doctrine of humours, quite often because the attributes ascribed to a plant or drug had been carefully 'cooked' to explain results that had already been discovered in practice, some very odd conclusions also emerged: salmon, for example, was at one time said to cause leprosy, for no other reason than that the *qualities* of salmon were akin to the qualities ascribed to the leper. This curious belief had its effects on rules of diet to the extent that salmon, a common food fish in the rivers of medieval England (not yet polluted by chemical waste), was sometimes expressly forbidden. In *Healths Improvement* Thomas Muffet says: '. . . hot salmon is counted unwholesome in England, and suspected as a leprous meal.'

This belief is obviously quite ancient: in the Scots Parliament in 1386 a regulation was made concerning bad pork and salmon, and the ingenious idea put forward that these could be given to lepers (presumably on the basis that the salmon could do lepers no more harm): 'Gif only man brings to the market corrupt swine or salmond to be sauld, they sll be taken by the Bailie and incontinent without ony question sall be sent to the lepper-folke; and gif there be no lepper–folke, they sall be destroyed alluterlie.'

There is even a tradition that the indentures of apprentices used to specify that the lads should not be given salmon too frequently because of the risk of leprosy. The Rev R. Polwhele, in his *History of Cornwall* (1806) says:

As this disease of leprosy is now extinct, it must have sprung from some cause which is . . . done away. The more prevailing notion is that the leprosy was generated by the eating of salmon too frequently, and at unseasonable times. That our forefathers thought so, is evident in covenants which I have seen in this county, and in Devon, stipulating that no apprentices or servants shall be obliged to dine on salmon more than once or twice a week.

According to Elihu Burritt, 'the learned blacksmith' from Connecticut, similar clauses were sometimes written into American apprentice indentures, apparently just as a slavish copy of older English documents, as there does not seem to have been any prejudice against salmon in New England in general. (*Walk from London to John o'Groats*, 1864.)

Some of the writers on 'humours' seem to have used the flexible nature of the theory to rationalize their own personal likes and dislikes. In *Klinike, or the Diet of the Diseased* (1633), James Hart, Doctor in Physicke, produces a respectable humoral background for most of his statements, but is inclined to wander off into rather personal diatribes—on cabbage, for instance:

> Cabbage is an evill nourishment . . . and ingenders melancholy . . . The Germans make also there a sallet of Cabbage small shred, with vinegar and oils, and all set about the dish with red-herrings, and hard-rosted eggs; the which who so is in love with, let him have his liking; and I thinke wee might spare our hard rosted eggs out of our sallets, and use them after a better manner.

Similarly, having said that shellfish 'ingender crude, viscous and phlegmaticke humours,' Hart expresses his real feelings about such food: '. . . prodigious gluttony hath now devised to feed upon the excrements of the earth, the slime and scum of the water, the superfluity of the woods, and the putrefaction of the sea; to wit, to feed on frogs, snails, mushrooms and oisters.'
Mushrooms come in for criticism elsewhere in the book:

> As concerning mushrooms, or Toad-stools, as they are commonly called, [they are] in small request here amongst us; howbeit in *France, Italy*, and adjacent countries . . . in no small esteeme. I advise therefore all our Gentrie, who travell into those forraigne countries, if they be wise, altogether to absteine from such excrements of the earth.

According to the French writer Louis Lemery, who published his *Treatise of Foods in General* many years later, around 1700, mushrooms and other fungi were regarded with considerable suspicion even in France at the time. He warns his readers to indulge in mushrooms only in moderation, and regards truffles, now such a delicacy, as only fit for feeding animals ('swine-bread').

On new and exotic fruits of the earth, Hart in particular was cautious, and inclined to suggest that the taste for these novelties would soon die out:

That out-landish root brought unto us from the *West-Indies*, called commonly *Potato* and by some *Batato*, is of the same nature and property [as skirret roots, a type of water-parsnip], but this pre-eminence it hath, that it is, according to the common proverb, *Farre fetcht and deare bought, and therefore good for Ladies*.

Nowhere is the flexibility of the Doctrine of Humours better illustrated than in the attitudes of various seventeenth-century writers to sugar and honey. Honey was of course the old-established sweetener, sanctified by centuries of use and the praise of the classical medical authors such as Aristotle and Galen. Sugar, which had up to about 1600 been extremely expensive, and only used for making luxury confectionery for the very rich, had fallen in price dramatically when the seventeenth-century trade with the East opened up, and was freely available for such dishes as fruit tarts and puddings.

One immediate result of this was that the teeth of the well-to-do who could afford to eat large quantities of the new sugary dishes, began to show rapid signs of decay, especially as the custom of cleaning the teeth was not very common. The courtiers, always the first with new fashions, were inevitably also the first to display the stigmata of excessive sweet-eating: a visitor to England in 1598, Paul Hentzner, who saw Queen Elizabeth arriving at the Royal Palace of Greenwich, remarked on her black teeth, 'a defect the English seem subject to, from their too great use of sugar'. (*A Journey Into England*, translated by Horace Walpole, 1757)

Hart also noticed the effects of sugar on the teeth, but his deductions from the humoral doctrine led him to the conclusion that sugar was almost entirely deleterious in its action:

Sugar being much used produceth dangerous effects in the body: as namely, the immoderate use thereof, as also sweet confections, and sugar-plummes, heateth the blood, ingendreth the *Iandise* [jaundice] *obstructions, cachexies* [sickness], *consumptions*, rotteth the teeth, maketh them look blacke; and withall, causeth many times a loathsome stinking breath.

Honey, on the other hand, Hart considered entirely harmless and beneficial. Lemery took the entirely opposite view—honey was of doubtful value, while sugar was a boon to mankind. He spends a good deal of space describing the contemporary methods of refining sugar, and how the juice boiled from the sugar canes is treated with whites of eggs and lime-water to remove impurities and make first grey 'Muscovade' sugar and then a white sugar. By contrast with this: 'Honey is no proper Food for persons of a hot and bilious Constitution; because it's soon inflamed in them, and readily turns to Choler.'

Thomas Muffet took the same line in *Healths Improvement* (1655): '. . . for whereas hony is hurtful to cholerick complexions, Sugar is incommodious or hurtful to none.' Muffet worked on the logical basis that, as sugar was a well-known preservative for fruit and similar food (it was used in some quantities even for meat preservation), it must have a similar protective effect on the human body. This argument was taken up by several later writers, including Frederick Slare, who wrote a curious book *A Vindication of Sugars against the Charge of Dr Willis, other Physicians and Common Prejudices* (1715) including the following deathless couplet on sugar:

> That which preserves Apples and Plumbs,
> Will also preserve Liver and Lungs.

Not that Dr Muffet's logic was always so easy to follow. He had a habit of noting down curious 'facts' with a charming disregard of dialectical sequence or credibility—for example, the theory that if ducks' eggs were hatched under a hen, they miraculously lost the fishy taste that normally characterizes them. Muffet, or 'that ever famous Thomas Muffet, Doctor in Physick,' as he modestly describes himself on the title page of his book on diet, subtitled 'or Rules Comprizing and Discovering the *Nature, Method,* and *Manner* of *Preparing* all sorts of Foods used in this Nation', was really an uncritical collector of any strange or wonderful scientific facts that came his way. His *Insectorum, sive Minimorum Animalium Theatrum* (Of Insects, or the Theatre of Little Animals) has the same charm and sympathy with his tiny characters as one later finds in Fabre, but some of his ideas about the lives of insects would be more suitable for fairy stories than for a book on natural history. This may have been why his name is perpetuated in the nursery rhyme that deals with an apocryphal meeting between his daughter and a representative of the *Opisthatheae*.

Similarly, on diet, his scientific views are strange, even for the time. However, he notes down a number of facts of interest as a reflection of the state of food production in the seventeenth century; for example: 'The Irishmen, like to *Plinies* Barbarians, have not yet so much wit as to make a Cheese of milk; and our Welshmen want cunning to make it well. French cheese in *Plinies* time tasted like a medicine, but now the Angelots of Normandy are counted restorative.'

He also had an interesting theory about the origins of meat-eating, that this was not a natural process, but forced on people because of the need to reduce the population of animals and birds that would otherwise eat all the available vegetable food:

> . . . albeit by their rites of religion the Egyptians were forbidden to eat eggs, or to kill for meat any living creature, yet necessity caused them to eat both, lest their corn should be devoured both in seed and blade, or they forced to do nothing else but to bury young rabbits and to squash eggs; perhaps upon the foresight of the like inconvenience, God appointed man to eat flesh and fish: least happly overflowing the earth by dayly increase, there should scarce be any food left for man. . .

One thing on which Muffet, Hart and Lemery agreed completely was that bread was the staff of life, and that the coarser kinds of bread were far more nourishing than white bread. Hart said:

> . . . And such as feed more freely on fish and flesh, and eate less bread, have not their flesh so firme as those who feed most on bread; besides, that oftentimes their breath smelleth strong . . . Bread made both of pease and beanes is hard of digestion, of a drying and astringent quality, yet very

strengthening; and well moistened is good to strengthen labouring people.

Muffet went even further, and insisted that white bread was more indigestible than wholemeal bread, as well as being less nourishing. Lemery adopted the same point of view, and explained this indigestible quality in white bread in terms of the texture of the loaf:

The less Bran you leave in the Wheat Flower, of which you make Bread, the . . . better tasted the bread will be; but on the other hand, 'tis harder of digestion, and heavier on the Stomach, because the small parts of the Flower unite so closely one with another, that there are hardly any pores left in them.

Whatever the dietitians might say, the general public wanted white bread, and as bread was such a large part of poorer people's diet throughout Europe until at least the late nineteenth century, perhaps they were the best judges. 'White' bread, in any case, was not what we should understand by the term now. Modern white flour is made by passing the wheat through rollers, which crush the centre of the grain to flour. The bran from the outside of the grain remains in small flat pieces which are nearly all sieved out, and unfortunately one of the actions of the rollers is to crush the wheatgerm, which is rather oily, into a small flat disc which is also sieved out with the bran, thus considerably reducing the vitamin and mineral content of the flour. Stone-grinding, which was the sole method of milling until the middle of the nineteenth century, ground the germ as finely as the flour, so that even when the meal was 'bolted' through fine linen cloths to sieve out the bran, the germ went through with the flour.

This had two effects: 'white' flour in early centuries was really creamy yellow, and the loaves made with such flour were inclined to be rather flatter and closer textured than our modern bread. Because such bread was in reality rather difficult to chew, especially without butter or any other food, bakers were tempted to use various devices to make the loaves whiter and more open in texture. In the country such devices were easy to detect, but in the towns bakers used alum as a raising agent and chalk, whiting, and sometimes even more dangerous materials like white lead, to improve the appearance of the loaf. This adulteration gradually got worse as time went on and the towns grew more populous—the bakers were less and less likely to be personally known to their customers. By the eighteenth century, when there had been a number of poor harvests and consequently inferior corn had to be used in the flour, some of the worst town white bread was probably just as adulterated as Smollett suggests in *Humphry Clinker:*

The bread I eat in London is a deleterious paste, mixed up with chalk, alum and bone-ashes; insipid to the taste and destructive to the constitution. The good people are not ignorant of this adulteration; but they prefer it to wholesome bread, because it is whiter than the meal of corn. Thus they sacrifice their taste and their health, and the lives of their tender infants, to a most absurd gratification of a misjudging eye; and the miller or the baker, is obliged to poison them and their families, in order to live by his profession.

But, as Smollett was forced to admit, even when the townsfolk suspected that their white bread was adulterated, they still preferred it to darker and perhaps more nutritious bread. Perhaps the real lesson is that the proponents of wholemeal and other darker breads containing bran do not in practice eat very much bread: those who have to depend on bread for a large part of their diet prefer it white. For the very poor, who were chronically under-fed and often acutely hungry, bread was often the only ingredient for a meal, and bread without butter, milk, or broth to help it down is quite difficult to eat. In medieval times, in particular, a mild degree of scurvy from shortage of vitamin C was almost universal among the mass of the population, and one of the first effects of scurvy is inflammation of the gums leading to loss of teeth. Imagine yourself eating tough wholemeal or rye bread with nothing but water to moisten it, and with a very inadequate set of teeth, and you will understand why people insisted on white bread even against the best advice from their 'betters'.

In the country conditions were a little better, if only because milk was available, and milk can provide not only an adequate amount of protein, but also minerals, fat, and vitamins A, B, D, and even C if the milk is drunk fairly soon after it has been produced. Old Parr, who lived to the age of 152 years and 9 months, existed and even thrived on a diet of 'sub-rancid cheese, and milk in every form, coarse and hard bread, and small drink, generally sour whey,' as William Harvey wrote in the post-mortem report on the old man, adding, 'On this sorry fare, but living in his home, free from care, did this poor man attain to such length of days'.

It seems likely, in fact, that Thomas Parr might have lived a little longer had he not been noted down as an interesting curiosity by the Earl of Arundel, who brought him to Court to show to Charles I. The combination of polluted London air and a sudden change of diet to the rich court food was too much for the aged body as Harvey said:

> . . . for one hitherto used to live on food unvaried in kind, and very simple in its nature, to be set at a table loaded with variety of viands, and tempted not only to eat more than wont, but to partake of strong drink, it must needs fall out that the functions of all the natural organs would become deranged.

The belief in the merits of such simple food was widespread, and there is a characteristic word-picture by the Rev Edward Boys Ellman (*Recollections of a Sussex Parson*) of

> an old man, Tom Eager, who always said that he was going to live to be as old as Methuselah; for he had found out that Methuselah had lived on bread and cheese. So nothing would persuade the old man during the last twenty years of his life to touch any other food. I cannot say what his age was at death but I fancy it was not quite ninety.

Among the more literate people there was a vogue for the 'simple life' prompted by the publication of various translations of *Discourses on the Simple Life* (Discorsi sulla vita sobria) by Luigi Cornaro, a Venetian nobleman who died in 1566 at the age of 98, having for about 50 years gradually cut down his daily intake of food until, near the end of his life, he was living on one egg, some milk, and 14 oz of wine per day (it was, of course, unthinkable in Venice at the time to abstain from wine, as the water was calculated to lead to a very short life if used as a beverage).

Cornaro does not seem to have had much influence on European dietary theories until long after his death, but from about the eighteenth century his name crops up constantly in dietary reform literature. Nietzsche noted sourly that people were still starving themselves to death on Cornaro's diet well into the nineteenth century.

4 The Pythagoreans

The last two or three decades of the eighteenth century witnessed perhaps a greater change in the conditions and flavour of life and thought than any other similar period in history. There was not just one revolution going on, but a whole system of intersecting revolutions, each one influencing the others, and all developing at once.

In France, the enormous political upheaval of the final triumph of radicalism tended to overshadow all the other changes, but in England the effects of these other influences, not forced into the black-and-white polarities of politics, were possibly even more profound because they were harder to detect at the time. The Industrial Revolution was creating not only all the evils of the industrial proletariat and the teeming slums of the new cities, but a new and articulate middle class, not dependent on the land and no longer satisfied with the tastes and occupations of the older country gentleman, but ready to investigate new social and intellectual pursuits.

For the readers, Smollett and Sterne had already begun to create the type of novel that depended upon a close and detailed account of middle-class lives, and Jane Austen continued the tradition with more skill and delicacy, turning out a product ideally suited to the aspiring families who gathered in the fashionable spas and holiday resorts. Coleridge and Wordsworth were converting poetry from a distant and philosophical commentary on the futility of human life, as in the work of Pope and Crabbe, to an emotional and direct observation of life and death among ordinary people—not without moralizing, of course, but in simple and comprehensible language.

For those with a scientific bent, there was the new *Encyclopaedia Britannica* (four editions between 1771 and 1815), which could tell the enquiring reader everything from the reasons for the great age of Methuselah to a recipe for making 'sal armoniac' from soot, salt, and the urine of cattle. In 1797 Nicholson began to publish the first scientific magazine, the *Journal of Natural Philosophy, Chemistry, and other Arts*, and new scientific societies were formed almost every year—the Linnean, Zoological, Geological, Astronomical and Horticultural Societies all date from this limited period of time around 1800. The Royal Institution, destined soon to become an important centre of scientific life in England, with such great experimenters as Davy and Faraday, was actually founded in 1800, and very shortly commenced its policy of promoting public lectures to spread the knowledge of science to interested laymen.

For those more concerned with social matters, Adam Smith had just finished formulating the real principles of economics, to rationalize the manifestly creaking system of exchange and taxation that was failing to meet the new needs of industrial society. Tom Paine proposed more drastic methods of reform, and although there were few actual supporters of his socialist views, he was widely read and discussed. Almost every town had either a Club for Constitutional Information or a Society of Friends of the People, where Paine's *Rights of Man* and similar books were publicly read and debated. In support of the most depressed class of the population, Mary Wollstonecraft published her book *A Vindication of the Rights of Women* in 1792, and although this shrewd and brilliantly-argued account of the wrongs of women did not succeed in doing much to help their lot, it was a colourful and widely-read symptom of the intellectual ferment of the period.

Into this world of change and questioning of accepted values, Mary Wollstonecraft's son-in-law, Shelley, dropped like a fox into a henhouse, chasing each colourful group of ideas to its logical limit and some way beyond. Gifted with a commanding appearance, an angelic power over words, and some ability to handle ideas, he set himself the task of reorganizing the world.

His pamphlet *The Necessity of Atheism*, though not par-

ticularly blasphemous or even anti-religious by modern standards, resulted in his expulsion from Oxford University. His
social pamphlets laid out in beautiful prose the outline of a
kind of romantic socialism that appealed strongly to the demo-
cratic ideals of Coleridge and similar writers. And among his
other prose writings are two important essays on diet—*A
Vindication of a Natural Diet* and *Essay on the Vegetable Diet*,
both putting forward the view that vegetarianism produced
'health and virtue' while animal foods promoted 'disease,
superstition and crime'. In his early poem 'Queen Mab' he
explores not only his new social ideas, but dietetic ones:

> . . . No longer now
> He slays the lamb that looks him in the face,
> And horribly devours his mangled flesh,
> Which still avenging nature's broken law,
> Kindled all putrid humours in his frame,
> All evil passions, and all vain belief,
> Hatred, despair, and loathing in his mind,
> The germs of misery, death, disease, and crime.

So effectively did Shelley establish his position as a radical
writer, despite his death at the age of thirty, that his books and
pamphlets influenced other thinkers long after. When a Shelley
Society was founded by Frederick J. Furnivall, the great
philologist and editor of early English literature, Bernard Shaw
was one of the first members, and announced on joining that he
himself was 'like Shelley, a socialist, atheist and vegetarian'.

However, Shelley's pamphlets were not the first considered
works on diet reform. In 1797 an anonymous book was published in Manchester, *On the Conduct of Man to Inferior
Animals*, which puts a complete case for vegetarianism from
humanitarian, health, and moral grounds. It opens its argument
boldly from the title page, which has a charming Bewick wood-
cut of a dying deer in the forest, captioned: 'It was late a playful
fawn, which skipping and bounding, awoke in the mind of
FEELING observers, a thousand tender emotions. The butcher's
knife hath laid low the delight of its fond dam, and the innocent
is stretched in gore on the ground.'

After a long introductory essay on the skills and intelligence of animals, designed to counter any arguments that these are 'lower creation' only fit for man's food, the author demolishes the idea that the conventional diet of flesh is a healthy one:

> Every animal except man makes choice of his food, with sagacity and readiness, while this image of God is incapable of distinguishing from that which is baneful and unwholesome, till after he has brought on himself infirmities, diseases, and torments which contribute to shorten the natural term of his existence.

To establish the true diet which man should follow, there is a chapter 'The Primeval State of Man examined, and Instances of frugivourous Habits adduced from History', in which we learn among other things that 'the ancient Arcadians lived on acorns, the Argives on peas, the Athenians on figs'—and then science is brought to bear on the subject, in the shape of a Dr Elliott, who decided that digestion was a form of fermentation, and that fermentation was of three kinds—*vinous*, when fruits, grains, and so on are converted to alcohol, *acetous*, when the same materials go a further step and are converted to vinegar, and *putrefaction*, when foodstuffs rot. Dr Elliott's argument was that fruits and vegetables could undergo all three processes (a fact well known to those who make home-made wines, which sometimes pass all too rapidly from the vinous stage to the later stages of vinegar or worse), but that meat, which does not ferment to make alcohol or vinegar, can only rot, and must therefore already have passed through the first two stages: 'Animal substances can only pass through the latter stage and therefore have probably already undergone the former.'

One oddity of this theory, admitted by the author, is that using the 'fermentation' criterion, milk must be a vegetable substance, because it can be fermented to alcohol or vinegar. He notes this as proof that milk and milk products are suitable food for man, even if meat is not.

An interesting detail of the book is the evidence it provides that the cure for scurvy was well known in the eighteenth century, even if the cause was still osbcure—this author, of course, blamed it on meat-eating:

> . . . the disease most common to this country is the scurvy. One finds a dash of it in almost every family, and in some the taint is very deep. A disease so general must have a general cause, and there is none so obvious as the great quantity of animal food devoured by the natives. As a proof that the scurvy arises from this cause, we are in possession of no remedy for that disease equal to the free use of fresh vegetables!

The last part of the book is an account of the long and healthy lives passed by those who avoided the temptation to eat animal food, such as George Broadbent of Dobcross, a small textile village near Saddleworth in Lancashire, who lived to the age of 98 on a diet of 'milk-meats' and home-grown vegetables, or the remarkable slimming diet of Thomas Wood, a miller of Billericay in Essex, who gave up all his normal food and substituted a single dish at 4–5 am and noon:

> This consisted of a pudding, of which he eat a pound and a half, made of three pints of skimmed milk poured boiling hot on a pound of sea-biscuit overnight, to which two eggs were added next morning and the whole boiled in a cloth . . . Finding this diet however too nutritious, and having grown fat during the use of it, he threw out the eggs and milk.

Wood finished his incredibly boring diet by using a daily 'pudding' of a pound of coarse flour and a pint of water boiled together, and lost about 150 lb.

At this period, of course, it was not difficult for the ordinary people to be vegetarian, or almost so. Only the luckiest families had meat more than a few times a year, unless they could snare a rabbit or bird. Even this became difficult as the land came more and more into Enclosures under a few rich landlords, and the Game Laws were enforced rigidly. Mantraps and spring guns were common deterrents to poaching, and only in the remote parts of the north of England and Scotland was there any real chance for the labourer to obtain much meat from the land.

In the south of England, as commons were enclosed so that keeping a cow became impossible, even milk and cheese were hard to come by, as milk on large farms would be converted immediately to butter and cheese for sale, and the buttermilk fed to pigs. Jonas Hanway, writing about Stevenage in Hertfordshire in 1767, said: 'The food of the poor is *good bread*, cheese, peas, and turnips in winter, with a little pork or other meat, when they can afford it; but from the high price of meat, it has not lately been within their reach. As to milk, they have hardly sufficient for their use.' (*Letters on the Importance of the Rising Generation*)

Sir Frederick Eden, in *The State of the Poor* (1797) shows that conditions were probably worse by the end of the century: his weekly food budget compiled from a labourer's family consisting of husband, wife and four children in Streatley, Berkshire, gives their consumption as:

8 half-peck loaves
2lb cheese
2lb butter
2lb sugar
2oz tea
$\frac{1}{2}$oz oatmeal
$\frac{1}{2}$lb bacon
2 pints milk

In the north of England milk was easier to get, and Eden's budget for a Westmorland family includes about 4 gallons of milk a week as compared with the two pints in the south, but meat was still a very rare dish for the working man—Eden estimated less than 12lb of meat *per year* for the average labourer's family.

In Scotland, milk and cheese were again fairly readily available; Smollett, in *Humphry Clinker*, gives a description of life in the Lowlands through the letters of his character Matthew Bramble:

The country people of North-Britain live chiefly on oat-meal, and milk, cheese, butter, and some garden-stuff, with now and then a pickled herring, by way of a delicacy; but flesh-meat they seldom or never taste; nor any kind of strong liquor; except two-penny, at times of uncommon festivity. Their breakfast is a kind of hasty-pudding, of oat-meal or pease-meal, eaten with milk. They have commonly pottage to dinner, composed of cale or cole, leeks, barley or big, and butter; and this is reinforced with bread and cheese, made of skimmed-milk. At night they sup on sowens or flummery of oat-meal. In a scarcity of oats, they use the meal of barley and pease, which is both nourishing and palatable. Some of them have potatoes; and you find parsnips in every peasant's garden.

Life was different for the gentlemen: compare Smollett's account of the labourer's diet with the country-house meals Mr Bramble ate himself in Scotland:

We make free with our landlord's mutton, which is excellent, his poultry-yard, his garden, his dairy, and his cellar . . . We have delicious salmon, pike, trout, perch, par, etc., at the door, for the taking. The Firth of Clyde, on the other side of the hill, supplies us with mullet, red and grey, cod, mackerel, whiting, and a variety of sea-fish, including the finest fresh herrings I ever tasted. We have sweet, juicy beef, and tolerable veal . . . and plenty of partridge, growse, heath-cock and other game . . .

The upper classes, in fact, ate a great deal too much meat, and it was no strange thing for an ordinary country clergyman to give a dinner that included 'a large Cod, a Chine of Mutton, some Soup, a Chicken Pye, Puddings and Roots, etc. Second course, Pidgeons and Asparagus. A Fillet of Veal with Mushrooms and high Sauce with it, rosted Sweetbreads, hot Lobster . . .' and so on to the sweets and wines. (*The Diary of a Country Parson*, The Reverend James Woodforde (1758–1781))

To the more refined members of such society, vegetarianism must have had immediate attractions. More books rapidly followed Shelley's pamphlets, and the Rev William Metcalfe compiled a long list of cases where overweight or ill patients had been brought back to a proper size and condition by a vegetarian diet (*Abstinence from the Flesh of Animals*, 1821), and

Sylvester Graham, in America, produced *Lectures on the Science of Human Life* in 1839. Graham had realized that the presentation of vegetarianism needed more sensational treatment than had been accorded it so far, and set out to satisfy this need. His book is a farrago of misinformation: 'a single pound of rice, absolutely contains more nutritious matter than two pounds and a half of best butchers' meat . . . Incredible as this may at first appear.' Incredible indeed. He combined the science fiction with the type of moral argument that had so attracted Shelley, and which has been the mainstay of food reform literature at all times: flesh foods lead to wickedness, vegetarian food to virtue. Graham's new twist to this theory led him to a remarkable piece of circular argument: if flesh-eating makes people wicked, and the Flood was caused by the extreme wickedness of the antediluvian population, therefore they must have been great meat-eaters. It follows from this that God disapproves of meat-eating, otherwise he would not have sent the Flood: 'The enormous wickedness and atrocious violence and outrages of mankind immediately preceding the flood, strongly indicate, if they do not prove, an excessive indulgence in animal food.'

Apart from such flourishes, one of Graham's main diet rules was the use of stone-ground wholewheat flour containing everything that had been in the grain. His reasons for this were largely religious: if God had not intended us to eat the bran, etc, he would not have provided them. However, as the cult of 'whole' flour continues to this day, it is pleasant to note that some health-food stores in America still call it 'Graham flour'.

Graham also started one of the first vegetarian magazines, *The Graham Journal of Health and Longevity*, which had a wide circulation in the USA, combining, as so many magazines of the kind do now, dietary matters with general articles on the Good Life (the *morally* Good Life, that is) and a certain vein of homespun philosophy borrowed to some extent from Benjamin Franklin's *Poor Richard's Almanac*.

By 1847 there were enough convinced vegetarians in England for the formation of the first Vegetarian Society in Manchester, supported by such eminent seekers after perfection as Francis

William Newman, younger brother of Cardinal Newman, and a man of such probity of thought that he had resigned his Fellowship at Balliol because of conscientious scruples about the efficacy of infant baptism. The Society was later joined by Anna Kingsford, a tireless (but occasionally tiresome) worker for a variety of causes—anti-vivisection, Hermetic Christianity and the Esoteric Christian Union—and author of *The Perfect Way in Diet*. Dr Kingsford was an excellent speaker and organizer, and did much to bring the principles and ethics of vegetarianism to the general public and the press, until her untimely death in 1888. Anna Kingsford's vegetarianism was strongly influenced by mysticism, and her own belief that abstention from meat was divinely ordered. In this she was similar to her better-known contemporary Annie Besant, who took up vegetarianism with a large number of other Indian influences when working out the principles of Theosophy—she later actually wrote a book called *Vegetarianism in the Light of Theosophy*, which harked back to Shelley's views that meat caused a lowering and coarsening of the spiritual nature, while an austere vegetable diet was the true food for mystics—which, of course, is true if the diet is austere enough to cause hallucinations (see pages 136–7). However, Dr Kingsford was a sound enough organizer to make sure that the vegetarian point of view was put in as many attractive ways as possible. Writers and speakers of many different fundamental beliefs were encouraged to support the cause and set out as many arguments for food reform as could be found.

For example, a popular speaker and writer was A. W. Duncan, a scientist who was also a convinced vegetarian, and quite capable of explaining the point, fairly new at the time, that a meatless diet could be just as nourishing as a conventional one. Even he could not resist a tendency to make the flesh creep with ominous sounding chemical jargon—'Flesh contains . . . excrementitious matter or compounds that result from the breaking down of the proteids; these are known as creatine, hypoxanthine, xanthine and carnine; they are but little removed from urea'. (*The Vegetarian Textbook*, ed. Albert Broadbent, 1903.)

An even better way of advertising the vegetarian cause was to make it clear that the diet was not 'weakening' or unsuitable for athletes. A very popular speaker on this theme was Eustace Miles, founder of the chain of vegetarian restaurants that carried his name, but, more important for propaganda purposes, Amateur Tennis and Racquets Champion for three consecutive years. F. D. Nawell, a keen long-distance cyclist, addressed the Manchester Physical-Health Culture Society in March 1902 to assure them that his strange diet could furnish all the energy needed by an athlete. He claimed that vegetarianism was an infallible specific against colds and published his speech later in an extended form as a pamphlet, *Colds—Their Cause and Natural Cure*. Nawell's specific against colds amounted to complete avoidance of fat from animal sources: 'I never take animal fat, greasy food, nor butter; they are not necessary; milk and nuts will supply all the fat the body needs . . .' (It is not quite clear from his pamphlet why the butterfat from milk was acceptable, but became taboo if separated out in the form of butter.)

He took space, however, to outline the conventional vegetarian views of the time as a method of achieving the sort of health needed by an athlete: 'As a distinction between brown and white bread I have christened it in my own home as 'substance' and 'shadow' and so on, but he had one piece of ritual which is curiously at odds with all the other 'natural diet' theories of the time: 'as fruits contain acid, they should never be eaten at the same meal as vegetables and salads, which contain alkalies, one fights against, and neutralises the beneficial properties of the other.'

Most of the dieticians in the Vegetarian Society or its fringes were by this time stating correctly that most fruits create *alkaline* conditions when digested (this point is considered in more detail in pages 81–2). However, although Nawell's pamphlet was published by the Vegetarian Society of Manchester, no one appears to have questioned this piece of unorthodoxy. As in so much food reform literature, if theories sounded plausible they were accepted without demur, and one feels that any carping insistence on proof, or reference to facts, would have been considered ill-mannered.

Humanitarianism was another popular platform from which
to promote vegetarianism, especially in England, with its long
tradition of sentimentality about animals. Many writers
followed Tolstoy in asking the pertinent question—what would
the effect be if the average meat-eater were required to slaughter
the animals for him- or herself? Some of the revelations about
the conditions in the Chicago stockyards and meat-packing
factories that emerged around 1906 made many people think
very seriously about avoiding meat, partly because of the
appalling cruelty in the abattoirs that had been revealed (a
point already made by Tolstoy, but ignored to a large extent—
perhaps because people in the West imagined that such things
happened only in Russia), but also for fear of eating infected
food from the filthy conditions, or taboo foods such as horse-
meat. *Punch* made a number of heavy-handed comments on the
revelations about the Meat Trust, such as the following:

> The Admiralty has directed that American tinned meat shall
> no longer be a compulsory ration in the British Navy. An
> appeal has now been received from Chicago that the products
> in question shall be retained as a punishment in view of the
> impending abolition of flogging.

Upton Sinclair, whose revelations of conditions in the meat-
packing industry in his novel *The Jungle* had started all this, was
not so flippant. His scarifying book did a great deal to speed up
the passing of the Pure Food laws in America. He himself, not
surprisingly after months of research in the stock-yards, abattoirs and packing factories of Chicago, reported that he lived
on a meatless diet for about three years after *The Jungle* was
completed.

It is pleasant to note, in passing, that at least one modern
group of vegetarians base their diet on humanitarian grounds—
the Vegetarian Feminists of America consider that all animals
are equal in their right to life, and the meat-eater is therefore
behaving to cattle and sheep exactly as men do when they
exploit women. Their slogan is 'Women, are you still *human*
chauvinists? The All-Compassionate feminist is a vegetarian!'

Sometimes the wish to avoid animal products led to some strange conclusions: when the *New York Evening Journal* published an editorial deriding the vegetarian movement, in 1906, Otto Carqué replied in a pamphlet called *The Folly of Meat-Eating*. Starting off with a fine topical flourish—'The recent labor troubles in the slaughterhouses and allied industries of this country have more than ever brought the question to the front, "Is meat a necessary article of diet?" . . .'—he went on to outline the usual reasons for vegetarianism (humanity to the animals, health, longevity, the deleterious effects of meat on the morals and intellectual powers of those who ate it, and so on). He then proceeded to push his argument against the use of animal products even further: he was opposed to manuring the soil with 'filth—animal, bird, or human excrements, rotten bones, dried blood, sewage, etc.' and wanted only artificial manures used, '. . . even the poorest soil can be wonderfully improved by mineral fertilizers'. It is amusing to imagine the effects of this proposal on the present generation of food reformers with their demands for organically-grown, chemical-free crops unsullied by the products of the giant fertilizer manufacturers, yet it is really just as logical as many of the arguments against other animal products.

A reason for vegetarianism that appears in many writings on the subject is the argument from design—the idea that it was possible to prove that man was designed as a fruit and vegetable eater, and not for catching or eating other animals. Many people drew up anatomical tables showing how closely man's teeth, stomach arrangements, and so on were allied to those of the vegetarian animals, and how different they were from those of the carnivores. Opinion seemed to be divided, even in vegetarian circles, on the question whether man was intended to eat cooked or uncooked food. This was not just a religious argument that we must do what God intended for us: one must remember that Darwin had only recently drawn the curtain from the vast design of evolution, and no one in late Victorian or Edwardian times could fail to be influenced in some way by the dramatic demonstration of the rise and fall of species and their adaptation to new methods of living and feeding.

In *The Animal Kingdom* (1827) Cuvier had already set out the arguments against man as a natural carnivore:

> Fruits, roots and other succulent parts of vegetables appear to be the natural food for man; his hands afford him a facility in gathering them; and his short and comparatively weak jaws, his short canine teeth not passing beyond the common line of the others, and his tuberculous cheek teeth would not permit him either to feed on herbage or devour flesh, unless these aliments were previously prepared by the culinary process.

Later vegetarian apologists also drew attention to the practical uselessness of man's canine teeth for catching other animals, and the fact that his molars were obviously adapted for dealing with roots and grains that needed a grinding action rather than the tearing required by meat.

One of the reasons for the great interest in this respect of comparative anatomy was that it provided a convincing counter to one of the commonest gibes at vegetarianism—the idea that a meatless diet was for weaklings, only suitable for sedentary men or women with servants to look after them, and that it could not possibly be adequate for manual workers or anyone else who depended upon muscle power. As has been said, vegetarians could point to members of their society such as Eustace Miles as examples of physical prowess, but the anatomical argument pointed to an even stronger and more athletic vegetarian than even Eustace Miles—the gorilla. Gorillas have almost exactly the same dental layout as human beings, and, allowing for their larger size, a very similar digestive system. Yet these agile and immensely powerful beasts kept themselves going very well on a diet of vines, wild celery, thistles, bamboo shoots and similar vegetable products.

Critics pointed out that gorillas in the zoos seemed to eat meat, but naturalists who had studied the animals in their native conditions were able to assure the doubters that this was probably the result of the unnatural confinement, as wild gorillas had never been seen to eat anything but plant life. This has been confirmed recently: a good summary of the evidence on meat-eating in the primates is included in Janet Barkas's book *The Vegetable Passion*, Routledge & Kegan Paul, 1975.)

Into this world of pamphlets and proselytizing, with its factions and arguments about minute details of diet, came two young men—one aged nineteen, the other aged twenty—who were destined to have far more effect on the world than any of the other food-reformers, but, because they were also vegetarians, also had a tremendous influence on the public image of the movement: Mohandas Kamamchand Gandhi and George Bernard Shaw.

Gandhi, curiously enough, had been brought up as a vegetarian, in the orthodox Bania caste, and as a teenager rebelled against this on the almost political ground that Indians ought to be able to eat meat just as the British did. As he said himself, he believed, at about fifteen years of age, that 'meat-eating was good, that it would make me strong and daring, and that, if the whole country took to meat-eating, the English could be overcome'. To young Indians in the 1880s, 'food reform' meant abandoning vegetarianism and embarking on the modern custom of meat-eating. However, when he was due to go to England to complete his law degree, his mother was so worried about the corrupt atmosphere in London ('Someone had told her that young men got lost in England. Someone else had said that they took to meat; and yet another that they could not live there without liquor') that he made her a vow that he would not touch wine, women or meat, and kept his vow for ever.

In England he felt entirely lost among the strange people and customs, and found it very difficult to find suitable meatless meals. Then he had a stroke of good fortune which could only have happened in London at the time:

> I would trot ten or twelve miles each day, go into a cheap restaurant and eat my fill of bread, but would never be satisfied. During these wanderings I once hit upon a vegetarian restaurant in Farringdon Street. The sight of it filled me with the same joy that a child feels on getting a thing after its own heart. Before I entered I noticed books for sale

exhibited under a glass window near the door. I saw among
them Salt's *Plea for Vegetarianism*. This I purchased for a
shilling and went straight to the dining room. This was my
first hearty meal since my arrival in England . . .

With all the enthusiasm that typifies a new convert, Gandhi
not only gave up his plans to bring meat-eating to India, but
set about the task of bringing vegetarianism to Britain. He
organized a Vegetarian Club in Bayswater, where he lodged,
and persuaded Dr Jonas Oldfield, then editor of *The Vegetarian*
magazine, to become president, and Sir Edwin Arnold vice-
president. Arnold must have seemed a particularly sympathetic
person to Gandhi—he was a noted Sanskrit scholar and had
spent many years in India teaching the language to British
officers, and had recently published *The Light of Asia*, a poetic
and widely-admired book on Buddhism and its relations to
Christianity. Gandhi himself acted as secretary and arranged
many lectures and discussions.

Oldfield, like Gandhi, tended to regard vegetarianism as a
method of chastening the body, and for both of them fasting
and avoidance of 'exciting' foods formed an important part of
the regime. After Gandhi left England, having been called to
the Bar, his diet became more and more ascetic, and rapidly
ceased to be based on health reasoning; rather it became an
active method of disciplining the body:

'Fasting and restriction in diet now played a more important
part in my life. Passion in man is generally co-existent with a
hankering after the pleasures of the palate . . .' he wrote in
later years, and also 'One should eat not in order to please
the palate, but just to keep the body going'.

In a sense, therefore, as his influence in the world grew
greater, and his doctrine of *ahiṃsā* or non-violence became
better known, his personal attitude to food began to colour the
popular idea of vegetarianism. The vegetarian tended to be
regarded as an ascetic, renouncing all the pleasures of the flesh,
and many people must have thought to themselves that vegetarianism was religiously and morally good, but far too difficult
a system for the ordinary man or woman. On the other hand,

those whose natural caste of mind was ascetic tended to take up vegetarianism just to be like Gandhi, forgetting that the Mahatma himself had pointed out that fasting and renunciation in themselves are useless without the mental and spiritual effort that must accompany them. Gandhi, like most religious leaders, realized that austerity in itself is a very cheap way of making yourself feel virtuous. Real virtue is harder to accomplish.

Even so, the Gandhian practice of rejecting all the pleasures of the table found a sympathetic response in many members of the vegetarian community who had been attracted to the system for ascetic reasons. Even before Gandhi arrived in London, Francis William Newman, then president of the Vegetarian Society, had written with approval of

> the late Mr George Dornbusch, of Threadneedle-Street, [who] went even beyond Vegetarianism. He not only abstained from all the received animal foods—from everything that had animal life, and from eggs, milk and its products, but from every form of vegetable grease and oil, from the chief vegetable spices, such as pepper and ginger, and emphatically from salt . . . (*Frasers Magazine*, February 1875)

Bernard Shaw seems to have come into vegetarianism mainly because it was one of the trendy things to do among the English intellectuals he admired and envied. He had been drawn to the original Fabians—Sidney and Beatrice Webb, Sydney Olivier, the Rev Stewart Headlam, and Annie Besant—and through their interest in diet reform to Henry S. Salt, author of the book that had revolutionized Gandhi's ideas. Shaw accepted the package that went with the intellectual life of the period— socialism, vegetarianism, rational dress, educational and penal reform, and so on—and, as a pugnacious and brilliant speaker, went on to lecture the world about any or all of these causes whenever he had the opportunity: 'I first caught the ear of the British public on a cart in Hyde Park, to the blaring of brass bands,' he wrote later in the preface to *Three Plays for Puritans*, 'and this not at all as a reluctant sacrifice of my instinct of privacy to political necessity, but because, like all dramatists and mimes of genuine vocation, I am a natural-born mountebank.'

While Shaw did not remove the image of peculiarity from the public view of the vegetarian, he did a tremendous amount to convince the public that it was an eminently healthy regime. Apart from the great age that he attained, there was the continuing evidence of his unflagging intellectual powers which remained when many of his contemporaries were only too obviously ready for retirement—three of his masterpieces, *Heartbreak House*, *Back to Methuselah*, and *Saint Joan*, were written when he was well over sixty, and he maintained his taste for lecturing the public until his nineties.

When he became a household word all over the globe, he found himself so overwhelmed with correspondence from admirers or writers who wished to take issue with him on one or other of his numerous theories that he had to resort to a set of printed replies on the most popular subjects. One of these, on 'Vegetarian Diet', gives a clear idea of his food habits towards the end of his life:

Mr Shaw's correspondents are reminded that current vegetarianism does not mean living wholly on vegetables. Vegetarians eat cheese, butter, honey, eggs, and, on occasions, cod liver oil.

On this diet, without tasting fish, flesh, or fowl, Mr Shaw has reached the age of 92 [1948] in as good condition as his meat-eating contemporaries . . .

Nevertheless Mr Shaw is of the opinion that his diet included an excess of protein. Until he was seventy he accumulated some poison that exploded every month or six weeks in a headache that blew it off and left him quite well after disabling him for a day. He tried every available treatment to get rid of the headaches: all quite unsuccessful . . . He now makes uncooked vegetables, chopped or grated, and their juices, with fruit, the staple of his diet, and finds it markedly better than the old high protein diet of beans, lentils and macaroni . . .

The cod liver oil mentioned in the list of 'vegetarian' foods strikes an odd note, and there was in fact no reason for Shaw to take the oil himself—his diet would have been quite adequate in vitamins A and D, the main components of value in fish liver oils. He did, however, have to take extracts of liver (not the oil) for anaemia, which began to affect him seriously in 1938, when he was 82. This is a common ailment with vegetarians who do not eat many eggs, and is due to deficiency in vitamin B_{12}, cobalamin. This vitamin is only found in animal foods, liver, kidneys, and clams being rich sources, and unfortunately cannot yet be synthesized in the laboratory. For those vegetarians who do not object to eggs, there is not much difficulty in getting enough of the vitamin: although they are not as rich in B_{12} as liver or kidneys, two eggs a day will supply all of the vitamin needed by the average person, even in the absence of any other animal food. If milk or cheese are also in the diet, one egg is probably enough. However, those who do not eat any animal foods may easily develop a disease known as Addisonian pernicious anaemia, as the vitamin is absent from all vegetable foods and even ordinary yeast, one of the better sources of the other B vitamins. There are now some special yeasts which are grown on media containing the vitamin, and these can be used as a source of the vitamin because they absorb quantities of B_{12} as they grow, but this does not really ease the situation of supplying the vitamin in the first place, except by using animal sources.

As the vitamin was only discovered in 1948, no one in 1938 was in a position to tell Shaw the easy way to cure his anaemia —to eat more eggs and cheese—but it was already known that liver and liver extract would rapidly end the disease, although nobody knew precisely why. Shaw was given liver extract and appears to have accepted the situation realistically, although he did try to minimize the 'animal' background of the treatment by referring to the extract as 'those chemicals'.

However, journalists found out the situation, and naturally considered it a good story that the Grand Old Man of vegetarianism was 'cheating' on his diet. Alexander Woolcott spread the story in America, and there was an immediate outbreak of fury in the American Vegetarian Party that their idol should have feet of liver extract. Symon Gould of the Party wrote letters to Shaw in such a fierce vein that one can only imagine that he would have preferred the playwright to die unsullied than to go on living a useful life with the help of animal food. Shaw finally wrote a long open letter to Gould in 1948 telling him bluntly not to exaggerate the benefits of vegetarianism and to keep the moral and religious claims for the diet in some sensible proportion. He also made the point which is unfortunately still valid—that a strict vegetarian diet without dairy foods can cost a lot of money to keep up, because of the need for nuts and similar rather expensive sources of protein to replace the animal protein: 'What you have to rub in,' wrote Shaw testily, 'Is that it is never cheap to live otherwise than as everybody else does, and that the so-called simple life is beyond the means of the poor.'

To distinguish the 'strict' vegetarian diet from the easier regime allowing dairy products, it became the custom to call the strict dieters *vegans* and the others *lacto-vegetarians*. This at last settled a tedious debate that had been drifting on almost from the first days of the Vegetarian Society, and to which Shaw referred in his printed comments.

In the magazine *The Nineteenth Century* for June 1879 Sir Henry Thompson, the eminent physician and expert on diet, had spread himself at tremendous length on the topic of the word vegetarian and how it was misused by those who ate milk and cheese, etc. The Vegetarian Society reeled under the shock, and then recruited John Mayor, Professor of Latin and Senior Fellow at St John's College, Cambridge, a noted lacto-vegetarian, to compose a reply. This finally appeared in 1889. If it really took ten years to write one feels that Mayor hardly deserved his professorship, as the reply was a garble of texts from classical literature on the subject of diet, all of which had been quoted many times before by far less eminent members of the Vegetarian Society. The word vegan finally settled the question.

Vegans run a serious risk of deficiency diseases owing to the difficulties of providing, with a vegetable diet, all the essential materials that the human body cannot synthesize for itself. Vitamin B_{12} is one of these, and vegans often get anaemia just as Shaw did. Other materials are the essential amino-acids, some of which are not included in very large amounts in the vegetable proteins in nuts and pulses, and vegans can suffer from a kind of kwashiorkor arising not from a gross shortage of protein, but from a lack of some of the essential building-blocks for it.

For this reason, and the sheer monotonousness of a vegan diet, the system is not very popular compared with lacto-vegetarianism. However, it has great attractions for those who object on aesthetic grounds to animals being involved in their food, and even more for those whose approach to diet is a search for asceticism. If the vegans wanted a patron saint, they might like to consider St Genevieve, the patroness of Paris, who, in the words of Thomas Muffet, might be said to have followed the vegan diet: 'St Genoveve, the holy maid of *Paris*, who . . . abstained wholly from flesh, because it is the mother of lust; she would eat no milk, because it is white bloud; she would eat no eggs, because they are nothing but liquid flesh.'

5 The Carnivores

Vegetarian literature tends to give the impression that all dietitians are on the side of abstinence, and only custom, ignorance and gluttony keep the activity of meat-eating going. This is, of course, a travesty of the facts. For every vegetarian pamphlet there was a corresponding essay on the value of meat in the diet, and it was usually just as closely argued. There is such delight, for pamphleteers, to be running against the crowd, that we tend to forget the theoreticians working away to prove that the crowd were right all the time.

The custom of not only eating meat, but eating very little else, had a strong following among the athletic class, particularly university rowing crews and similar groups whose lives were dedicated to the one great pointless effort. 'Training' usually meant not only abstention from smoking and similar weakening habits, but the consumption of large amounts of protein food. The diet of the athlete, in fact, included the two great essentials of any convincing diet, sacrifice and ritual, and it was therefore treated seriously by large sections of the population. In *The Adventures of Mr Verdant Green* (1853) 'Cuthbert Bede' (Edward Bradley) pokes fun at the training fetishes of the Oxford boat clubs: '. . . the Brasenose bow had been seen with a cigar in his mouth, and also eating pastry in Hall—things shocking in themselves, and quite contrary to all training principles.'

For some reason the meat had to be underdone: 'It seemed a *sine qua non* with the gentleman who superintended the training for the boat-races, that his pupils should daily devour beef-steaks which had merely looked at the fire.'

Some of this lore had been handed down for generations, some of it came from books such as *The Art of Invigorating and Prolonging Life by Food, Clothes, Air, Exercise, Wine, Sleep, Etc.* (1821), a catchily-titled work by William Kitchiner, a doctor with considerable influence on the nineteenth-century dietetic scene. Kitchiner was particularly interested in two aspects of training—sport and singing. He realized, perhaps earlier than anyone else, that professional singing is a branch of athletics, and that a singer who is going to master the breath control and develop the chest and diaphragm muscles to give a good performance must be trained and fed exactly as an athlete is.

His diet for athletic training is Spartan in the extreme:

. . . they are directed to eat Beef or Mutton—rather *under* than over-done, and without either Seasoning or Sauce . . . *Broils* are preferred to either *Roasts* or *Boils*—and stale Bread or Biscuit.

Neither Veal — Lamb — Pork — Fish — Milk — Butter Cheese — Puddings — Pastry — or Vegetables are allowed.

Which amounts to a diet of underdone meat and dry stale bread.

Thomas Parry, a later physician, carried this tradition on into his diets for everyday life. In his book *On Diet, with its Influence on Man* (1844) he offers advice on suitable food for all classes of occupation:

On the Diet of a Labourer, or Man dependent upon Labour
On the Diet of the Light Mechanic
On the Diet of the Active Professional Man
On the Appropriate Diet of the Sinecurist
On the Diet of a Gentleman
On the Diet of Females
On Dietary for Intellectual Attainment

It soon emerges that Dr Parry had his quirky points. Vegetables obviously figure in a very low place in his table of values:

If the roots, stalks, and leaves of vegetables be used, the preference should be given first to the farinaceous roots, as

the potatoe; then to the sweet roots, as carrots and parsnips;
stalks and leaves should be used but sparingly, and then only
as condiments to meat and corn.

In fact, the phrase 'the roots, stalks, and leaves of vegetables'
begins to occur quite often, almost as a kind of malediction,
and it emerges that Dr Parry had a great dislike of the Dutch,
who, by improving the art of gardening and growing vegetables,
had increased their use. 'Gardening' itself becomes a sort of
swearword, and any other process or food introduced by the
Dutch, or even merely popular with them, is sure to invite a
storm of vituperation. Pork, for example—although pigs were
bred and eaten all over Europe, the Dutch had meddled with
their breeding and feeding: '. . . the multiplication of this
animal has been much increased since the introduction of
gardening from the Netherlands.' Therefore, by a process of
logic that is almost endearingly tortuous, this interference by
the Dutch made the pig unfit for food: '. . . in those districts,
and in those classes of men where the pig makes a chief article
of diet, tubercle in all its forms of scrophule and consumption,
and inflammations in the forms of eruptions, sore legs, bad
eyes, and abscesses, must prevail.'

Gin was another Dutch invention which had undoubtedly
caused a great deal of havoc among the poorer classes in
England, and this gave Dr Parry the opportunity to link all
his pet hates together in a comprehensive curse: 'Roots, leaves,
swine's flesh and gin, worthy compeers!'

Another bane was the use of hops in beer, another invention
of the Dutch in Parry's eyes (although hops had been in use in
English beer since the fifteenth century). He shows, in a remarkable passage, that hops were necessary in Dutch beer
because of the detrimental effects of their diet of pork and
vegetables:

And now we come to an exposition, why bitters came to be
used in diet, when the Dutch had sent us beasts' food to eat,
and the natural consequence was experienced in stomach-
pains, cholics, and all the catalogue of gastric miseries which
men relieved as well as they could by hot spices, spirits,

aether, foetid gums &c. . . . the introduction of bitters into the diet was, then, from the same people from whom we receive the garden-food, so calculated to pain, irritate, and injury the stomach, experience having taught them its use upon their own badly nourished bodies.

Not that Parry objected to ale, or un-hopped beer. In the chapter on the diet of a labourer, he recommends a daily ration of ale sufficient to raise the spirits of any working man: 'It should be good vinous stuff: it need not have the exquisite flavour of tokay, burgundy, madeira, or port; but it might and ought to have all the good mirth-making qualities of them all, without any ill, narcotic, deadening or impoisoning tendency.'

The upper classes, of course, could have something better than ale, and Dr Parry's use of the word 'exhilarate' for the raising of the spirits with alcohol gives a rather humorous picture of his 'professional man' at leisure:

The active professional man *should invariably exhilarate daily*, and always, if possible, with wine. This should always be done *after* the business of the day; and although, by exhilaration, I neither imply drunkenness, intoxication, nor any approach to the known term muddling, or maudling, yet this duty (exhilaration) should always be deferred till after business.

No doubt Parry's fellow doctors and lawyers suppressed their natural instinct to teetotalism and steeled themselves to do their duty by exhilarating themselves with wine, however distasteful this seemed.

His diet, apart from the necessary alcohol, resolves itself to bread and beef or mutton. Pork was taboo, fish would cause diseases of the skin, and vegetables were an invention of the Devil, or the Dutch:

Made dishes of vegetables: these are all flatulent, disposed to originate cholic pains and cravings of the stomach, and make great demands for brandy and hot spice. For those reasons, they may be left as standing examples of misdirected skill, or they may be given to those animals for whom the materials (vegetable roots, leaves, and stalks) are naturally destined.

A diet corresponding to Parry's recommendations was actually followed for a long period by a resident of Birkenhead called Bernard Moncriff, who left a complete record of his experiment in a book entitled *The Philosophy of the Stomach*, or *An Exclusively Animal Diet* (*Without any Vegetable or Condiment Whatever*) *is the Most Wholesome and Fit for Man* (1856). Taking his lead from Cornaro (see pages 36–7) he decided to limit his meals to cold roast beef, and originally also two quarts of milk ('good country milk'), the yolk of one egg, and some sweet almonds, as his daily ration of food and drink. In six months, he tells us, he had become much healthier and had lost 20lb from his original 154lb (which, according to a modern table of heights and weights, is about 12lb overweight for his declared height of 5ft 5in). Having maintained the diet for the full six months, Moncriff decided it was too rich, and eliminated the egg, almonds, and half the milk.

Some of his conclusions are extremely interesting: on this restricted diet he perspired very little despite regular exercise, and found that he needed little more fluid than the pint of milk provided. On the other hand, if he ventured to eat bread or potatoes, he became thirsty, and his intake of fluids increased greatly. After about a year on this monotonous diet, he found that he had lost the taste for almost all highly-flavoured food and drink—wines, beer, coffee, tea, and 'salt, pepper, mustard, vinegar, apples, pears, and some of the most fashionable "fish-sauces" which happened to be in my possession. Even honey and sugar had lost much of their attraction for my palate'.

The immediate impression of this diet is that it would rapidly lead to scurvy, because of the lack of vitamin C. However, the pint of milk, unpasteurized as it would have been at the time, would provide the bare minimum of the vitamin to keep scurvy away, and if the beef were not too overdone there might be traces of the vitamin in this too.

This trace vitamin in meat is very important for societies like that of the Eskimos, where fresh fruit and vegetables used to be almost unknown for most of the year, and raw or frozen seal and whale meat was the only source of food. Vilhjalmur Stefansson, the famous arctic explorer, lived for twelve months on the Eskimo diet of meat and fat only, and reported that he remained perfectly fit, never suffered from indigestion or constipation, and could carry out a heavy programme of physical work. As, by 1928, he had spent ten winters and thirteen summers north of the Arctic Circle, living mostly on the same food as the Eskimos, he was able to show that not only is their diet quite adequate to maintain health, but that it is also suitable for other races—it had previously been suggested by several writers that Eskimos had a different type of metabolism from that of more southerly peoples, which allowed them to live on a diet that would not be adequate for 'normal' people. Stefansson showed that, on the contrary, the Eskimo diet was very sound for anyone living in their climate, regardless of race.

However, while all these individual and isolated experiments and theories were being tried and developed, the greatest single contribution to nineteenth-century nutrition science was being worked out in Giessen, Upper Hesse, by Baron Justus von Liebig, one of the foremost chemists of his time. From about 1822 to 1838, he was concerned with the theoretical chemistry of the period. However, he became interested in the chemistry of plant and animal growth, and in thirty-five years of research laid the foundations of most of our modern knowledge of plant growth, fertilizers, and the principles of nutrition, sweeping aside the mass of conjecture and folklore about food and producing for the first time a set of theories that could be weighed and tested against the facts.

While his interest in the sciences of life started in 1838, it was a rather loosely worded commission from the British Association that really gave his studies impetus. In 1837 they had passed the following resolution: 'Professor Liebig was requested to prepare a Report on the present state of our knowledge in regard to Isomeric Bodies. He was also requested to prepare a Report on the state of Organic Chemistry and Organic Analysis.'

Liebig seems to have taken the 'request' as a challenge to produce something absolutely new in the field of organic chemistry, an account of the way in which plants were able to take very simple mineral ingredients from the soil and convert them into all the complicated vegetable products—starch, cellulose, proteins, and so on—needed for animal nutrition. This research was published in Germany and England in 1840 as *Chemistry in its Applications to Agriculture and Physiology*.

Always interested in the commercial side of his work, Liebig actually invented and put on the market the first 'chemical manure', based on his researches. It was not a success, for a variety of reasons—while it contained potash and phosphates, as do all good modern fertilizers, it had too little nitrogen to suit any plants but beans and peas. A stronger reason for its failure was the fact that the large-scale production of chemicals was in its infancy in 1840, so Liebig's ingredients were likely to cost more than the equivalent amount of organic manure from dung or compost.

However, intellectually, Liebig's ideas swept through Europe as a revelation. His work struck a decisive blow against the old theory that 'life could only proceed from life', or that plants not only needed living seeds to start them, but could only grow on material such as plant waste that had once itself been alive. Liebig's fertilizers based on purely mineral sources of potassium, phosphates, lime and ammonia proved triumphantly that plants could be grown with simple inorganic salts, plus water and the carbon dioxide in the air.

About the same time his friend and colleague Wöhler, working at Göttingen University, showed for the first time that an 'organic' substance, urea, which had previously been known only as a waste product of animal and human digestion, could be made from simple mineral materials. This was another blow to the 'vitalism' theory, and impressed the nineteenth-century intellectuals in a way that few chemical discoveries do today. Liebig and Wöhler are not to blame, of course, for the two directions in which their work was extended beyond its real relevance. In the history of ideas, their work became the basis for a lot of rather sterile mechanistic theory that every aspect of human life could be reduced to a few simple chemical equations, an attitude which held up physiology and psychology for decades, and in the history of agriculture, the indiscriminate use of mineral fertilizers without humus or fibre led to the 'dust-bowl' conditions of many large modern farms—farmers, having embraced Liebig's theories uncritically, are now gradually learning to modify them and give the structure of the soil the respect it deserves.

Having laid the foundations of a science of plant nutrition, Liebig left the practical agriculturalists to put his ideas into practice, and turned his attention to the needs of animals, including man. By 1842 he had produced a major work dealing with all aspects of the subject, *The Chemistry of Animals*. In this he classified foods for the first time into energy sources, the 'carbonaceous foods' as he called them (carbohydrates and fats, in modern terms), body-building sources ('nitrogenous foods', corresponding to proteins), and the various mineral components that were necessary for the production and renewal of bones and teeth. He wrote a book in 1847 that dealt in even more detail with the 'nitrogenous foods', *Chemical Researches on Meat and its Preparation for Food*.

As with the researches on plant growth, his theories on food had an enormous impact. Not only chemists and physiologists read and discussed his work, but amateur scientists, journalists, and even housewives became familiar with Liebig's ideas and his classification of foods. 'Carbonaceous' and 'nitrogenous' foods were as widely known in the 1850s as calories and vitamins are now. For instance, a series of didactic articles in *The Ladies' Treasury*, one of the first women's magazines, called 'My Lady-Help and What She Taught Me', constantly refers to Liebig and his theories when describing the principles of cooking. The lady-help, Miss Severn (a lady so omnisciently patronizing that she would have had any normal mistress of the house reaching for the meat-cleaver long before the lessons were completed), was depicted as a great enthusiast for scientific cookery:

My father, being a working chemist, knew well all about the

necessary amount of carbon, nitrogen, and other matters
which go to build up a healthy body . . .

The great chemist Liebig, years before he died, said that
meat should be put into boiling water, and then the temperature lowered . . .

Mrs Beeton, in the first edition of her *Cookery Book*, refers
to the same recommendation:

. . . Liebig, the highest authority on all matters connected
with the chemistry of food, has shown that meat so treated
[boiled from cold water] loses most of its most nutritious
constituents. 'If the flesh,' says the great chemist, 'be introduced into the boiler when the water is in a state of brisk
ebullition, and if the boiling be kept up for a few minutes,
and the pot then placed in a warm place, so that the temperature of the water is kept at 158° to 165°, we have the
united conditions for giving the flesh the qualities which best
fit it for being eaten.'

In passing, it may be interesting to note, from an episode in
'My Lady-Help', the type of diet common among the middle-
classes in Liebig's time. This is a family crisis: Mrs Newton,
the mistress, rushes into the kitchen with alarming news: 'My
husband has brought two clients of his, and is anxious to show
them some hospitality. They leave by the six o'clock train; it
is now nearly three. What can be got for their dinner that may
be quickly done?' With only three hours to prepare a hurried
snack, Miss Severn does not panic: 'Salmon and caper sauce,
lamb and mint sauce, mutton cutlets, young carrots, and
potatoes, will not be a bad impromptu dinner, for they can't
expect anything else, except sweets . . . We can have stewed
rhubarb and macaroni cheese.'

With eating on this scale when even an 'impromptu' dinner
demanded fish, two choices of meat, and a savoury, it is not
surprising that Liebig spent so much time studying the nutritional value of meat, nor that his books should have been read
with such interest all over Europe. It is unfortunate that the
series of articles never got round to Miss Severn's idea of a *big*

meal—perhaps there would not have been space in the magazine for a description.

Although most of Liebig's theories were correct, one of his main ideas about meat-eating was not. Liebig believed that muscles were physically used up during heavy work, and that therefore large amounts of protein were needed to replace this loss. He also believed that the only suitable nutrient to make the replacement was actual muscle protein, in other words meat. So while he recognized that plants contained 'nitrogenous food' (which he called 'vegetable fibrine' and 'vegetable albumen'), of use for some body-building purposes, he decided that only meat would serve to make up the losses due to work.

Such a theory was accepted almost uncritically, partly because of the great (and deserved) reputation of Liebig and his English translator and disciple, Lyon Playfair, but also because the middle-class Victorians were great meat-eaters by choice, and were quite pleased to be told that their diet was also scientifically approved. Liebig's theories were constantly advanced as an argument against vegetarianism, despite the evidence that a great many people in all parts of the world appeared to live quite healthily without meat. It was not until two respected researchers, Fick and Wislicenus of Zurich, started to question the theory that scientists began to doubt it, and even then they had to perform the rather spectacular experiment of living on a diet entirely free of nitrogenous food while climbing the 6,500ft Faulhorn. Despite the intense physical effort, they were able to show that their muscles had not wasted away even in the absence of meat.

The general public took longer to convince, and indeed it is doubtful whether many people in the West today believe that they can manage without meat. Athletes still train on diets exactly like those described in *Verdant Green*, eating as much as 2lb a day of underdone meat, and only enough vegetables and fruit to keep up their vitamin levels. It has been shown, in fact, that despite all the money and time spent on athletes' training, some of them go into their events suffering from vitamin B_1 deficiency because of the shortage of vegetables in their training diet.

Even among food reformers, the belief in meat as something magically special persists: Miss Barbara Cartland has been known to say, apropos of virility 'If every woman fed her husband two pounds of good red meat every day there wouldn't be any need for all these dirty films.'

When a TV company asked the inhabitants of a small Yorkshire village to switch from meat to soya protein for a week, as an experiment in modern nutrition, the response showed the expected mixture of interest and prejudice. The vicar's wife agreed to co-operate with the test except for the one day of her parents' fortieth wedding anniversary, when anything short of the traditional Yorkshire 'meat tea' would be unthinkable. The church warden was more forthright:

> I think a man who is going to do a decent day's work and earn a living wage can't do without meat. I fail to see that anything else will keep up his stamina. I think it's all very, very foolish.
>
> I don't believe in all this monkeying about with people's diets by statisticians and the like who have nothing better to do. (*The Times*, 15 August 1975)

It emerged, by a strange coincidence, that the outspoken church warden was also a wholesale butcher, but no doubt his words would find an echo in many Yorkshire hearts even without his specialized interest. There is a Yorkshire saying that no meal is complete without 'something that's drawn breath' on the table.

Even for the diet of invalids, there was, and still is, a strong prejudice that meat must somehow be stuffed into the patient if life is to be preserved. Mrs Beeton suggests 'a nourishing food can be made of raw beef, scraped free from fibre, seasoned with a little pepper and salt, and served as sandwiches between thin bread and butter,' and, for sick children, possibly the most revolting mixture in any cookery book—the same raw beef with 'a little sugar or jam instead of the savoury flavouring'.

Another favourite invalid food was beef tea, a kind of bouillon made by putting a pound of beef into a quart of cold water and then bringing the mixture to the boil slowly. Alexis

Soyer, the great chef, even found it worth his while to compose a recipe for a 'savoury beef tea', so popular was the beverage for invalids.

Liebig, during his experiments on meat, had of course examined beef tea, and came to the quite correct conclusion that, as normally prepared, it contained very little nourishment, and definitely no body-building powers. The 'nitrogenous food' in beef tea consists mainly of gelatin, and as this protein contains none of the essential amino-acids (see pp 155–66) it is of very little use to the metabolism. Liebig knew nothing of the amino-acids, but he knew from experiment that gelatin was somehow 'deficient' and had no tissue-forming qualities. He decided therefore that the virtues of beef-tea must arise from the mineral constituents of the meat, extracted during the long boiling, and also from the boost that it could give to jaded appetites, often encouraging invalids to eat something nourishing even if it were of little use itself.

This appetizing quality had been known for some years, and the nineteenth-century nutritionists had called the unknown material created in meat by cooking 'osmazome':

Osmazome . . . communicates to animal substances that peculiar flavour called savoury . . . The flesh of game and of full-grown animals contains the largest proportion of it. Vauquelin has discovered it in the mushroom, and Chevalier and Lassaigne assert that it exists in some plants belonging to the family of the Chenopodiae. (*Food and its Influence on Health and Disease*, Matthew Truman, 1842)

There seems little doubt that osmazome is a mixture of amino-acids released by the breakdown of the meat protein. One of the most savoury flavourings is the salt of one of these amino-acids, monosodium glutamate, which exists in large amounts in cooked meat and in some vegetable preparations. For example, soy sauce, made from fermented soya beans, contains so much monosodium glutamate that it can be used to give the illusion of cooked meat in rice dishes containing little or none. This is the basis of its use in Chinese and Japanese cookery. Monosodium glutamate is also added to processed cooked meats, savoury soups, and so on. It is rather comic to find food reformers who object to this latter practice as 'putting chemicals into food' still using soy sauce, or the Japanese miso and tamari that are staples of the macrobiotic diet, all of which contain far more monosodium glutamate than any other packaged foods.

During his work on beef-tea, Liebig also found that he could concentrate the extract into a stable form suitable for keeping. It only needed hot water to make a satisfactory beef-tea. Again anxious to make some commercial use of his discoveries, he set up a company to make 'Liebig's Extract of Meat' or *Extractum Carnis*. This time he had a success on his hands. The Argentinian and other South American meat producers, in the 1850s, were just beginning to feel the effects of over production of beef. Meat-canning had been carried on for some years, but this was not an ideal solution to their problems, because the process was not very efficient until 1870 at the earliest, and some of the canned meat turned out in the 1840–60 period was so badly preserved that the public were justifiably scared of it.

Ships' crews, an obvious market for corned beef and mutton as an alternative to the notorious 'salt junk' they had eaten before, were often struck down with food poisoning by the canned meat. (This was basically because the principles of food preservation were not discovered until the time of Pasteur, and the manufacturers, trying to make large economical packs of meat, had not realized that the centres of the cans could not be sterilized by external heating.) Sailors developed a folklore all their own about the mysterious contents of the cans: corned mutton was called Fanny Adams, after a girl whose dismembered body had been thrown into a river at Alton, near Portsmouth, in 1812, and Harriet Lane, similarly butchered by a murderer called Wainwright, was believed to have a posthumous existence in the form of naval rations.

Liebig's discovery of the meat extract process was therefore welcomed by the meat producers: his product had every commercial attraction. It made perishable beef into a product that was almost indefinitely stable, so that gluts of meat could be turned into extract for several seasons ahead; the volume of the meat was reduced without loss in value, thus saving packing and shipping costs, and, though this was not so widely advertised, almost any part of the animal could be used in the process. The Fray Bentos producers and Liebig formed a company to make his beef extract in Uruguay in 1864.

As Liebig's Extract of Meat, or Lemco, or *Extractum Carnis*, the product was an immediate success, probably helped by the claims that 1lb of the extract contained the 'concentrated essence' of 36lb of beef. Most people probably believed that this meant *all* the properties of the beef, including the protein and body-building components. Liebig obviously knew that this was not the case, but he seems to have restrained his natural scientific distaste for a half-truth very successfully.

As Bovril, Oxo, and so on, similar extracts have continued to the present day, relying on the simple, and provable, appetizing qualities of the product to provide the advertising appeal. Liebig's Extract of Meat Co. Ltd. is still retained as a working company registration by the Brooke Bond Oxo Company Ltd.

One peculiar aspect of meat-eating in England arose around 1867, when, owing to a cattle epidemic in the previous year, beef was in very short supply and therefore expensive. Serious efforts were made to encourage the eating of horse-meat, which was called *chevaline* to make it appear a little more attractive. Horse-meat had already been sold in Paris, and there was a famous *Banquet Hippophagique* in 1864, when all the meat dishes were prepared from horse-flesh, which was copied in the Langham Hotel in London in 1868 by The Society for the Propagation of Horse Flesh as an Article of Food. *Punch*, in the punning style of the period, wanted to know why horse-radish and horse-chestnuts had been omitted from the menu, not to mention *Pie*-bald, and a little later (and a little more wittily) produced two definitions:

HIPPOPHAGY (from *hippos*, a horse, and *phago*, I eat), 'The eating of horseflesh'.
HYPOCRISY (from *hippos*, a horse, and *crisis*, a judgment), 'Saying horse-flesh is very good'.

In April 1869 at Cambridge a nine-year old donkey was fattened and butchered, and served up at the table of the Master of Trinity. The experiment does not seem to have started a fashion, or even to have been repeated. Perhaps the remarks from Oxford about cannibalism had something to do with this.

6 Wise Men from the West

Dietary systems are like religions—if they are to catch the attention of the public, they must have a definite ritual connected with them, and preferably some element of sacrifice and chastening of the senses. Tell people in the Western world that they ought to have a more varied diet and simply eat less than they do at present (which would solve most of their problems) and you will not find more than a handful of followers, and the media will ignore you. Say, on the other hand, that they must eat 10lb of stewed rhubarb without sugar every day, or that they may only have coffee if they put in salt and cider vinegar instead of sugar and milk, or that they must never eat eggs at the same meal as bacon, and your dietary system will be in every women's magazine and Sunday supplement, and thousands of people will try it—for a day or so.

It is not surprising, therefore, that just as the modern art of publicity was developed in the USA, so were some of the most bizarre and widely-followed dietary systems. Almost as soon as the American nation had got itself organized so that most of the population had enough food, Cassandras arose to tell the Americans just how disastrous their food habits were.

One of the first people to realize the supreme importance of ritual in dieting, and to provide a system strange enough to give it an outlet, was Horace Fletcher. In many ways an unusual man to have left his mark (and his name) on the history of dietetics, Fletcher was a highly-skilled New England businessman. He was born in Lawrence, Massachusetts, in 1849, and

by the time he was thirty had made a sizeable fortune manu-
facturing printing ink, a vital commodity for the explosive
growth of literacy in the 1870s and '80s. He also catered for
the expanding social life of New England by importing silk
from China and Japan.

In his forties, he was well enough known as a sound businessman to be invited to take over the management of the New
Orleans Opera House, then going through one of its regular
financial crises, and helped to make the fine French colonial
building the centre of the city's cultural life.

Then, in 1895, Fletcher had a traumatic experience. An
insurance company refused to accept him as a life risk because
he was 50lb overweight—not an unusual condition for businessmen in the sybaritic atmosphere of New Orleans in the '90s.
However, Fletcher worried about it. He accepted his weight as
a challenge, set himself to study the methods of other noted
weight-shifters such as Banting, and finally evolved a diet that
was conventional in most ways, but included as a new ingredient
The Ritual. Every mouthful had to be chewed until it was
completely broken down to a soft paste, so as to give the
stomach as little subsequent work as possible.

How Fletcher arrived at the idea of this faintly disgusting
practice it is hard to say. He gave many lectures and interviews
to explain his method, being blessed with a popular and
cheerful style that pleased newspaper editors, and he wrote a
number of books—*The New Glutton or Epicure* and *The A.B.-Z.
of our own Nutrition*, both published in 1903, and the rousingly
boastful *Fletcherism: What it is; or How I Became Young at
Sixty* of 1913—but most of his explanations seem to come back
to the simple apodictic virtue of chewing for its own sake, and
the rather revolting physiological explanations that he offers
are rationalizations after the event. V. H. Mottram, the distinguished nutritional expert, called Fletcherism 'one of the
saner food fads', because at least the prolonged chewing could
do no harm, and for most people accustomed to wolfing down
their food it could do a great deal of good.

What Fletcher had really discovered, of course, was that the
interminable chewing not only took a great deal of time, and

thus physically cut down the amount of food that could be swallowed, but also removed any pleasure from eating at all, by fatiguing the sense of taste to the point where the most savoury mouthful was usually reduced to the texture and flavour-appeal of wet newspaper. H. D. Renner in *The Origin of Food Habits* (1944), points out the 'sacrifice' element in Fletcherism and the corresponding feeling of virtue when the sacrifice has been made:

> To men of even normal senses it is just appalling to treat a savoury bite in such a manner that by the time it is ready to be swallowed it has, apparently, acquired qualities which we are accustomed to associate with sawdust. For there are so many people who, by nature, are insensitive that it is almost of no importance to them what kind of food they eat. These people are the ones predestined to become victims of a fad like Fletcherism. But there is also the power of the human will, able to overcome whatever stands in its way, and it is this power that may have enabled Fletcher and his devotees to practise their ideas . . .

No wonder Fletcher and his followers lost weight: their meals must have been incredibly boring occasions. 'We Fletcherised raw carrots and peanuts till our jaws ached,' recalled one South African food reformer, describing the methods she had tried and discarded in her search for the True Way. The idea of incessant chewing as an aid to health spread to circles where Fletcher's own name was unknown, and chewing every mouthful thirty-two or fifty times passed into the repertoire of common catch-phrases. In Aldous Huxley's *Antic Hay*, for example:

> 'Bite, bite, bite,' he said. 'Thirty-two times.' And he opened and shut his mouth as fast as he could, so that his teeth clicked against one another with a little dry, bony noise. 'Every mouthful thirty-two times. That's what Mr Gladstone said. And surely Mr Gladstone'—he rattled his sharp, white, teeth again—'Surely Mr Gladstone should know.'

Whether thirty-two, or fifty, or a hundred, the number of chews is quite arbitrary. The physiologists have measured the number of bites necessary to reduce various foods to a reasonable state for swallowing, and find that it varies from one bite for soft bread to as many as a hundred for a stringy bit of ham in a sandwich. Chewing the soft bread fifty times more than it needs will not assist digestion, but it will make the bread so wearying and nauseating that there will be no temptation to eat much of it.

Fletcher himself seems to have taken his status as a dietetic guru very lightly. He was of course pleased with his loss of weight and his good health (he celebrated his fiftieth birthday in 1899 by riding 200 miles on a bicycle) but was never bigoted about food. Sometimes he would experiment: as one visitor recorded in 1900: 'I met Mr Horace Fletcher, the author and traveller . . . He had been living a week on baked potatoes for experimental reasons when I met him, and without experiencing any morbid sensations: a more perfect specimen of physical health I never gazed upon.' On other occasions he indulged himself—one of his biographers records charmingly that 'he could often be publicly seen taking second helpings of turkey'.

He used his wealth and public name to encourage scientific work on nutrition, subsidizing research at Harvard and Yale, and during the 1914–18 war he went to Belgium and lent his undoubted talent for organization to welfare work, trying to ensure that the limited supplies of food were used in the best possible way. In the end, long hours of work and constant travelling under wartime conditions wore down even Horace Fletcher's ebullient good health (he was approaching seventy) and he died in 1919, just too soon to see food reform and slimming cures expand from a hobby for the literate few to a public obsession.

In the upheaval of the 'twenties, preconceived ideas about food were swept aside or stood on their heads, along with pre-war standards of social correctness, fashion, or morals. People were in a mood to be adventurous after the austerities of the war, and the war itself had opened the eyes of many of them to the rich possibilities for a new way of living. Most of the serving soldiers had been outside their own countries (or even away from their home towns) for the first time in their lives, and they had been forced to admit that the strange customs and unfamiliar foods of the foreigner might have some sense to them. At home, particularly in Europe, food shortages had made the housewife experiment with new cuts of meat and different vegetables, and had even forced the conservative males to try the new foods, or go hungry.

As well as a desire for change and a break from the old, stodgy pre-war foods, there was a passion for slimming. Fashion played a key role in food habits. The comfortable matronly plumpness that had looked distinguished in Edwardian costume or portrayed by Charles Dana Gibson appeared simply *fat* in the 'twenties look. Bright colours, short shirts and shapeless tops made plump women look rather like gaily-painted barrels, and it was no longer enough to rely on a slim ankle when most of the rest of the leg was on show. The cult of casual clothes for men showed up the fatties almost as much. *Punch* of the period is full of caricatures of businessmen 'with full round belly' trying to look athletic in Fair-Isle sweaters and plus-fours.

Every newspaper and women's magazine ran its column on dieting, and gossips exchanged 'cures' as they had been used to exchange experiences of the servant problem in pre-war days. Some of the information was sensible, some crazy, and much of it downright dangerous, but as few people kept to the diets for very long or very strictly, not much harm was done.

Most would-be slimmers followed the course that Sinclair Lewis parodied in *Babbitt*—talking about it—

'Folks don't give enough attention to this matter of dieting. Now I think—Course a man ought to have a good meal after the day's work, but it would be a good thing for both of us if we took lighter lunches.'

'But Georgie, here at home I always do have a light lunch . . .'

And then, like Babbitt, most people yielded to the lunchtime temptation:

That morning he had advocated lighter lunches and now he ordered nothing but English mutton chop, radishes, pease, deep-dish apple pie, a bit of cheese, and a pot of coffee with cream, adding, as he did invariably, 'And uh—Oh, you might give me an order of French fried potatoes.'

For the weak-willed Babbitts there sprang up batteries of health clinics, fruitarian cures and reformed diet nursing homes, where rich Americans could pay to be starved. The regimes were usually based on the models of the best German spas such as Baden, where minimal diets were combined with drinking the mineral water. In America, lacking the supply of foul-tasting waters, the clinics added their touch of magic by concentrating on strange and wonderful dietary systems.

The simplest of these diets, and without any doubt the least expensive to arrange, was that of Dr Edward Hooker Dewey, a physician of Meadville, Pennsylvania. He claimed that a prolonged fast was by far the best way to cure almost all diseases, and even for the well food should not be eaten earlier in the day than noon, and preferably not till nightfall. His book *The No-Breakfast Plan and the Fasting Cure* (1900) is full of accounts of patients who lived for periods up to fifty days with only water as their nourishment, and during this period of grace were cured of diphtheria, diabetes, cancer, and a host of other ills.

Dr Dewey is a lively writer, and the case-histories have real dramatic effect as he builds up the tension to the thirty-fifth or forty-second day, or whenever the moment of truth is to be revealed. The reader expects that on the great day, every case will end with the complete cure of the patient, the triumphant call for food after the long fast will mark complete recovery. Unfortunately, it appears that a number of the patients died, but Dr Dewey counted these cases as successes for his method if they died quietly 'with the mind perfectly clear to the last,' as he often puts it. Obviously a quiet and dignified end is what most of us would wish when it becomes inevitable, but as a recommendation for the dietary system it seems an anticlimax.

On the other hand, one must set Dr Dewey's methods in the context of conventional medicine at the time. He started his medical work, he tells us, during the Civil War, when whiskey was often the only item of *materia medica* available—anaesthetic, tonic, and antiseptic all in one. After the war the use of whiskey continued, and patients were often dosed with alcoholized milk, usually one pint of whiskey to one quart of milk, each day. This mixture (and quantity) was given even to the dangerously ill and to small children. Dewey apparently gave up this barbaric treatment when one of his own children developed diphtheria, and the mixture of whiskey and milk made the child so wretched that the father in Dewey overruled the doctor. He was surprised to find that although the child took nothing but water for some days, it gradually recovered, and at last asked for food spontaneously. Such an experience obviously weighed heavily with him, and he carried on to evangelize the virtues of fasting for the rest of his professional life.

Almost as simple, fruitarian diets were very popular, and as almost all the clients in the clinics were overstuffed with pies and cakes, and probably a little short of vitamin C, a few days of such a diet would take off a pound or two of surplus weight and improve the condition of the skin. Even if the customers did not feel better, the health clinics had a highly-developed double-talk to explain any symptoms—basically, if you felt good, that was the effect of the cure, and if you felt terrible, that was a symptom of your body 'throwing off poisons'.

'Distressing symptoms occur during the Grape Diet, through the poisons which have been stirred up by the action of the grape and thrown into the blood stream . . .' writes Mrs Johanna Brandt, a great proponent of this particular cure (*The Grape Cure*, 1930). She then goes on to describe the 'distressing symptoms' with a completeness and attention to detail which I shall not, out of consideration for the reader, repeat except for this summary:

To the inexperienced person it is disconcerting to find strange and new symptoms of disease developing under the

Grape Cure. He needs someone with experience to explain to him that poisons which have been locked up in the system for many years have broken loose and are running riot in the blood. Hence that unusual rise of temperature, that eruption on the skin, those splitting headaches, those attacks of retching and purging, that discharge of mucus, those undue sweatings. The anxious mind of the patient should be set at rest by the assurance that all these are highly favorable symptoms of the process of purification being carried out internally—*positively prove that he is still vital enough to respond to the treatment.* The avenues of excretion—the bowels, kidneys, lungs and skin—are still in good working order. Let him then closely examine the stools, the urine, the perspiration, and let him *rejoice* with the appearance of every new evidence that Nature is still able to cast out the poisons that have been dislodged by the magical action of the grape.

And in such happy pursuits many clients of the health clinics spent their time, acquiring the kind of self-knowledge that comes from a really detailed study of one's physiological processes. Mrs Brandt did not, of course, intend her Grape Cure solely for slimming or losing weight: she recommended it wholeheartedly for cancer, arthritis, gall-stones, cataract, diabetes, tuberculosis, syphilis, catarrh, and stomach ulcers. Actually though, for those who want to lose weight, I can recommend Mrs Brandt's book as an ideal method. It is not necessary to take up the diet—any detailed reading of more than a few pages of the book will cause a complete aversion to food for several hours.

Other fruitarian diets abounded, and were warmly recommended by the fruit growers, if not by the medical profession. Blackberries were recommended for diarrhoea, oranges for arthritis, and carrots for tuberculosis. More recently there has been a revival of the Grapefruit Diet, with the new twist that there was a magic ingredient in grapefruit that made the body burn up fat. Obviously if anyone can manage to eat nothing but grapefruit for several days, they will achieve a temporary loss of weight, but otherwise the system did very little for anybody except the grapefruit growers and importers.

The supposed scientific basis of most of these diets is an attempt to reduce the 'acidity' of the diet. Meat, starchy foods, sugar, and most of the other foodstuffs disliked by food reformers—so runs the theory—are changed into acid by the body, and this acid gives rise to indigestion, heartburn, stomach ulcers, constipation and diarrhoea, and almost every other physical, mental, or moral illness, if one believed everything written about fruit cures. Vegetables and fruit, on the other hand, produce alkaline conditions and neutralize the acid, thus reversing the ominous process.

There is some truth in this theory, despite the apparent anomaly that sharp-tasting fruits like oranges and lemons could be alkaline when digested. The organic acids in fruit and vegetables—citric acid in oranges, lemons and other citrus fruit, pineapple, tomatoes and raspberries, malic acid in apples, plums, quinces and tomatoes, malonic acid in beetroot, and so on—taste very acid in the mouth, and would corrode metals just like other acids, but they are oxidized so rapidly in the digestion that no trace of acidity remains after a very short time, while the mild alkalis also present in the fruit are left to exercise a beneficial effect. On the other hand, like most of nutritional theory once it has got into the hands of food faddists, the acid/alkali story has been very much over-simplified.

Some fruits like cranberries and bilberries, for example, contain an organic material called benzoic acid, which is just as natural as the others, but apparently of no use to the human body. When we eat cranberry sauce, for example, the benzoic acid is passed undigested to the liver, which processes it to the less harmful hippuric acid before it is excreted. Other foods— tea, cocoa, rhubarb, spinach, sorrel, pepper, and so on— contain substantial amounts of oxalic acid. In the small amounts that we normally consume, in tea, for example, this acid can be oxidized and disposed of, but if we eat too much at a time it is poisonous, either depositing 'gravel' in the kidneys or, in larger doses, causing death. People have died through trying to supplement their green vegetable diet with rhubarb leaves.

Other natural organic acids are just not digested by the body, and therefore tend to increase acidity. Ironically, in view of the fantastic claims made for the Grape Cure, the tartaric acid in grapes is one of these indigestible materials, and for a diet designed to combat acidity no worse fruit could be found. It seems quite likely that the 'distressing symptoms' of the Grape Cure were in fact the inevitable effects of large amounts of tartaric acid in the system, especially among those patients who followed Mrs Brandt's advice and ate up to 8lb of grapes per day.

Fruit diets, as has been said, probably did some good for the average American businessman of the early 1900s, accustomed to a diet rich in starchy pastries, cream, sugar, and particularly excessive amounts of protein in the form of meat and cheese. Even in 1875 Francis William Newman, President of the British Vegetarian Society, had commented on the cult of meat-eating in America: 'In the American Union physical abundance has long reached the lowest class; butcher's meat is eaten as often as they please by the population in town and country, and no part of the English race is so unhealthy as they.' (*Frasers Magazine*, February 1875)

However, it must be admitted that the diet of the British businessman seemed to differ very little from that of his American counterpart. *Dagonet* (George R. Sims) writing in *The Referee* for 13 September 1880, satirized the traditional fare on his side of the Atlantic:

> The ordinary English meal consists of slabs of raw meat, slabs of heavy pudding, wedges of new bread, and heaps of semi-boiled vegetables. No wonder we riot and howl and kick our wives, and go in for coarse pleasures after such a Zoological Garden system of feeding.

In the circumstances, it is odd to find that one particular diet recommended *only* meat: perhaps the attraction was that it allowed the dieters to indulge themselves in plenty of steak, while at the same time keeping the necessary elements of ritual and sacrifice by cutting out everything else. Unlike the system of Moncriff mentioned earlier (p 62), which would have been monotonous but at least palatable, the diet of Dr J. H. Salisbury was Spartan to say the least, consisting of 1lb of minced beef and four pints of hot water per day, the beef to be rolled into little balls and lightly cooked on a griddle, or occasionally boiled. Neither Dr Salisbury's reasons for this diet, nor those of his disciple Elma Stuart, who wrote *What Must I Do to Get Well?* and provided the diet as the unlikely answer, are very clear: he was bitterly opposed to starches and sugar, pulses and grains, but does not say what his objection was to fruit. Perhaps it was mainly that fruit was the panacea for rival dietitians, and Salisbury was determined to be different. Whatever the basis, the diet, conceived around 1885, was in use in various clinics in the USA well into the 'thirties and possibly even longer: I have seen references to it in dietetic literature of the 1950s that suggest it had only recently been entirely abandoned.

What finally killed these older diets was not the fact that they did not work—if this book contains any message at all, the message must be that failure is the last reason why anyone gives up an essentially magical custom—but the fact that they were too easy to understand, and the mystique was lost. The science of nutrition, between 1900 and 1940, provided a whole new shining set of magical symbols—vitamins, minerals, essential amino-acids—and the mass-media were quick to publicize each new discovery and make the words at least common property. The pseudo-nutritionists were quick off the mark to weave fresh theories out of the exciting new raw materials, which gave such scope for blinding the public with science, for a brand-new magic with Words of Power.

7 Science Fiction

At the present time, when the climate of public opinion has turned distinctly chilly about science, it is difficult to appreciate the sense of adventure and excitement conveyed by scientific discovery in the early years of this century. We think of the thousands of new materials introduced by chemists every year, and wonder sourly how many of them are going to cause cancer, or pollution, or the deaths of fish and birds. In 1900 every new material—aluminium, chromium, synthetic drugs and dyestuffs —was evidence that man had at last achieved mastery over nature, and that he could repair her omissions by his own ingenuity. We think of radioactivity as a constant major threat, and X-rays as a minor one, but to our grandfathers they were the first fascinating insight into an invisible world of rays and particles with infinite possibilities. It is not surprising, then, that while most modern food reformers turn their backs firmly on science and technology, and try to persuade us to leave nature to her own devices, earlier writers tumbled over themselves to prove that their particular diet made use of all the latest scientific wonders.

Those of us who have seen thousands of gallons of milk poured away because it was contaminated with radioactive strontium from a nuclear power station, or know that leukaemia can be caused by even a slight rise in the background radiation from other radioactive materials, must wonder about the motives of those who travelled to spas in Austria where radioactive uranium and thorium salts are present in the water. As far as they were concerned, the mysterious rays must do something, and the idea that the something might be harm did not occur to them or their medical advisers. In fact they were among the first cases of radiation sickness ever reported.

For those who could not afford to travel to the spas, there was *Pesqui's Vin Urané* ('being a compound of old Bordeaux wine . . . to which the following elements have been added: azotate of uranium, pepsine, and other appropriate elements'). As the uranium nitrate content was only 0.02 per cent, and the wine cost (in 1909) eight shillings (40p) a bottle—when reasonably good claret could be had, un-uranated for less than two shillings (10p)—there was not really very much danger that Dr Pesqui's customers could afford enough uranium to do themselves much harm.

Soon the cult of the new radiations as a cure-all became general, and nutritionists would hardly deign to look at a new diet system unless it could be shown that the food had mysterious electrical powers or occult rays emanating from it. Dr Robert Bell, MD, FRFPS, etc., of the Psycho-Therapeutic Society Ltd of London, published a book *Dietetics and Hygienics Versus Disease* (1910) in which he proved that uncooked food was the best way to health because it was radioactive, and the radiation formed a magical 'Vitalising Agent': 'It has recently been demonstrated by actual experiment that all fruits and seeds also contain radio-active elements when in an uncooked condition . . .' Apparently the mysterious power did not survive cooking. Some fruits had even more interesting powers: '. . . by means of a recently constructed recording instrument of acute sensitiveness it has been proved that each section of an orange is sufficiently charged with electricity to cause a galvanometer to record this fact.'

By a strange coincidence, there is an advertisement on the inside cover of Dr Bell's book for Eugene Christian's Natural Curative Foods, with the claim, 'These Foods contain the pure elements of nutrition in their natural form. The radio-active property of the grain is preserved in them, the vital principle not being destroyed by fire.'

As so often happens, there was partial truth in Dr Bell's claims. Many foods are radioactive because they pick up and concentrate natural or artificial radioactive elements, either in their basic structure or in the mineral salts that exist in most vegetable food. For example, radioactive carbon, carbon-14, is produced in the upper atmosphere by cosmic rays striking atoms of nitrogen in the air, and sooner or later all this carbon comes down to earth and becomes incorporated in every type of organic material, animal and vegetable.

Fortunately carbon-14 gives off its particles so slowly that it can do very little harm to the cells in which it gets involved, or the tissues round them—indeed, because this slow radiation goes on for thousands of years, the amount of carbon-14 in prehistoric materials can be measured and used to calculate the exact age of the samples.

Another widespread radioactive element is potassium-40, which is picked up by plants from the minerals in the soil, along with ordinary potash compounds. When we eat the plants we also absorb the potassium-40 into our cells, and this could be harmful if the radioactive material stayed there permanently. However, the turnover of potassium in the body is so rapid that any particular atoms are likely to be in and out within a few days.

Apart from these two materials, the only other radioactive material that could have been detected in Dr Bell's 'fruits and seeds' would have been the 'classic' elements uranium, thorium, and radium. From this point of view, 1910 was a Golden Age, with no artificial radioactive elements floating around. Not a single atom had been split, and the idea of nuclear energy was still hidden in the almost incomprehensible mathematical formulae of an ex-patents examiner called Albert Einstein.

Actually, the germ of grains and the kernels of nuts seem to have some mechanism for concentrating the tiny amounts of these radioactive materials that occur in the soil. Wheatgerm tends to be more radioactive than the rest of the plant, and brazil nuts in particular are so efficient at picking up these heavy metals that 1oz of the nuts contains almost as much uranium, thorium, and radium as the whole body of the average human being (unless, of course, they work in a uranium mine).

Perhaps the most ironic thing about Dr Bell's cult of 'radio-active' foods is that he also claimed that they were the only reliable way to cure cancer (*Cancer: Its Cause and Treatment Without Operation*, 1903), yet this book and the method are still quoted by nature-cure enthusiasts who are bitterly opposed to the use of radioactive materials such as radium or cobalt-60 in the medical treatment of the disease. No doubt they believe that there is a 'natural' radioactivity that is beneficial, and completely different from the nasty artificial radioactivity used by orthodox doctors. For example, Cyril Scott wrote a book specifically titled *Victory Over Cancer—Without Radium or Surgery* (1969) and devoted a scathing chapter to the futility of the use of radium, X-rays, and other radiations. He then included an equally long chapter recommending Dr Bell's methods warmly. Here again we have an interesting example of the ability of many writers on 'natural' medicine and food to believe two mutually contradictory theories at the same time.

As a final word on radioactivity in food, it must be said (though hardly emphasized, for post-Hiroshima readers) that however right Dr Bell may have been about the existence of radioactivity in certain foods, his claims that these radiations were some kind of 'vitalising principle' were tragically wrong.

The electrical and radiation cults waned in the 'twenties and 'thirties, partly because, as with any trendy idea, they grew old-fashioned, but mostly because there was a far more interesting development for anyone concerned with food—the steady uncovering of the vitamins.

Lunin, an obscure experimenter in Estonia, had discovered in 1880 that mice died if fed on an artificial mixture containing all the then known constituents of milk. He concluded that 'a natural food such as milk must therefore contain besides these known principal ingredients small quantities of unknown substances essential to life'. Spurred on by the discovery by Sir Frederick Gowland Hopkins and others, around 1906, of two actual examples of these 'unknown substances', vitamin research became the main study in nutrition and an unfailing source of new magic substances to excite the food reformers.

Hopkins, in Cambridge University, Eijkman, feeding polished and unpolished rice to chickens in Java, and McCollum with his enthusiastic young team of scientists at the Wisconsin

Department of Agricultural Chemistry, in a remarkable piece of joint research that straddled the world, had isolated what McCollum called 'fat-soluble A' and 'water-soluble B' by 1912. The work must have been rather more laborious than looking for a needle in a haystack—the only way of telling whether any particular fraction of the food contained the elusive vitamins was to go through lengthy feeding trials with animals, and see whether they developed deficiency diseases or not, and the actual amounts of the materials sought were less than 1 part in 10,000 of the food. In 1907 Holst and Frolich, in Oslo, showed that a similar substance present in tiny amounts in food made the difference between health and scurvy, but failed to find the actual material of vitamin C.

Into this picture of painstaking effort, lengthy trials, and analysis of tiny quantities of food, suddenly plunged a brash young Polish biologist called Casimir Funk. With what may be considered incredible far-sightedness (but what must have seemed to Hopkins and the other workers unforgivable gall) he coined the name *vitamine* for the new magic material. In 1914 he wrote the first book on *The Vitamines* in which he not only appropriated the work on 'fat-soluble A' and 'water-soluble B', but declared roundly that it was now certain that beriberi, pellagra, scurvy and possibly rickets were caused by the lack in the diet of 'special substances which are of the nature of organic bases, which we will call vitamines'. This book made vitamins news, not only in scientific circles, but in newspapers and magazines, and during the next few years further vitamin discoveries quickly became part of general dietetic folklore.

By the 'thirties, when most of the vitamins had been isolated and assigned to their true purpose in diet, public interest in scientific feeding was intense. Newspapers ran articles on the dietetic views of sportsmen, actresses, politicians and other experts. The *Morning Post* in 1936 ran a long series of enquiries into the food of the famous, and spent much space discussing the anomaly that quarter-miler A. G. K. Brown ate a great deal of fish during training, while the great Jesse Owens declared, 'If there is one thing more than another that I avoid, it is fish'. In the same year A. P. Herbert, then writing a weekly humorous article for *Punch*, devoted two of his spots in quick succession to a fairly serious discussion of diet—although one of them included a couplet from an unfinished poem:

> There are three vitamins, not four:
> I have no doubt there will be more . . .

and the suggestion:

> It is difficult to imagine an Act of Parliament *compelling* the people to eat a proper amount of the right vitamins. But we may be driven to the remedy suggested long ago in these columns—a system of licences and penal taxes for those who sell non-vitaminiferous foods. The grocer would be 'Licensed to retail bacon, tea, coffee, cocoa, sugar and jam.' And indigestion might be made a capital offence.

The second article, on bread, would cause some surprise even in present-day *Punch*—tables of protein, fat, carbohydrates and calories, comparisons of nutritional data (on bread and potatoes) prepared by the British Medical Association and a League of Nations Committee on the Problem of Nutrition, and so on —but was apparently of intense interest to the *Punch* reader of the time. True, APH was, as so often, tendentious and wrongheaded, and perhaps sensing this E. V. Knox, the editor, added a little tailpiece to the piece:

> The Editor of Punch declines to take a particle
> Of responsibility for the statements in the foregoing article.
> The reader may agree with it or he possibly may doubt it,
> But I don't intend to enter into correspondence about it.

The trouble was, APH had been reading Dr W. H. Hay, and Dr Hay represents one of the oustanding examples of creators of science fiction in dietetics. Other theories come and go and are mercifully forgotten, but Dr Hay's theories have a habit of turning up in various guises in books on diet and food reform even to this day, possibly because of their bold sweep of imagination, completely untrammelled by fact.

William Howard Hay, MD, ran the Sun-Diet Sanatorium for the benefit of suffering humanity, or at any rate that section of suffering humanity that could raise the substantial fees. He evolved, as part of his treatment, a dietetic theory of much complexity, and explained this at length in his book *Diet and Food* (1934). Complex or not, if one could believe Dr Hay, the diet was well worth adopting:

> . . . if the normal food habits intended for man were fully understood and practiced in every case, this would be a very much better world than it is, for disease would practically disappear, crime would subside, insanity would be scarcely if at all in evidence, and there would be less, very much less, imbecility and physical and mental imperfection in our wonderful country . . .

One thing the diet could not apparently eliminate was Dr Hay's passion for phrases like 'our wonderful country'. In his books America is never America, it is always wonderful if not glorious. The world is scarcely ever the world, but this *old* world, or this old ball of clay. His treatments never simply cured—they filled the patients with Vim, Pep, Vigor, and a host of other qualities that sound like brand names for detergents.

There were two cornerstones of the Hay Diet: the magic sixteen elements and the combinations of foods. The sixteen elements were oxygen, hydrogen, carbon, calcium, potassium, nitrogen, phosphorus, chlorine, sulphur, fluorine, magnesium, sodium, iron, silicon, manganese and iodine. Apart from being essential to human nutrition, Dr Hay saw these as the ideal fertilizer for plants—he spends a great deal of space on an experiment comparing plant growth in 'volcanic rocks' containing the sixteen elements, normal barnyard manure, and a commercial fertilizer referred to as '3-part fertilizer' which was presumably an ordinary artificial product based on nitrogen, phosphates and potash. Needless to say, the volcanic rocks came out on top, beating the despised artificial fertilizer and even the barnyard manure, which is rather surprising when one considers Dr Hay's unbounded admiration for natural 'organic' methods of plant growing, as expressed elsewhere in his books.

Of course, there is nothing basically untrue about the list of elements quoted. They all exist in the body, and in fact they were probably adopted by Dr Hay from one of those rather ghoulish analyses, popular around the turn of the century, that reduced the human body to its component parts, rather like a sample of soil. Popular science magazines had great fun translating these analyses into homely equivalents—the human body contained twelve gallons of water, enough carbon to make a small pile of coke, iron for three penny nails, and so on.

The list, as Dr Hay gave it, is incomplete—zinc and copper are at least as important as manganese, and human beings also need traces of cobalt, molybdenum, selenium, chromium, nickel, tin and vanadium—but this is a minor point. The real hocus-pocus starts when Dr Hay starts to list the foods we must eat to keep up our supply of the precious elements.

For example, the innocent biochemist sees that the reason why oxygen and hydrogen come first in the list is that the body is largely composed of water, and these are the elements that make up water. Similarly carbon occurs in every scrap of the food we eat—indeed, fats, starches, sugar, and most vegetables consist of very little else but carbon, hydrogen and oxygen. So, if we eat or drink at all, we must get enough of these three elements, apart from the oxygen we breathe in from the air.

Not so, say the Hay dieters. Oxygen comes from mint, parsley, rhubarb, and tomatoes. Exclusively, according to E. Gilbert Oakley, a follower of Dr Hay and at one time editor of *Here's Health*. This must make life difficult for people who live in countries where these four plants do not grow, but perhaps they have a special Divine dispensation not to need oxygen. Similarly, according to the theory, carbon is only obtainable from apples, dates, grapes, lentils, and tomatoes, and hydrogen from melons, some other fruit, and vegetables without starch. Those who take the diet seriously, and conscientiously eat these specified foods to obtain their oxygen, hydrogen and carbon remind one of people living on the shore of a huge lake of sweet fresh water, but buying their drinking water in half-pint bottles.

Some items in the list are correct, of course, if only by accident. Proteins, for example, are the main source of nitrogen for the body, and the Hay diet specifies beans, cheese, fish, peanuts, and milk, all rich in protein and more acceptable to some people than meat, the other important source.

Other items are irrelevant, such as the lists of foods containing chlorine and silicon. Chlorine, according to Dr Hay, is obtainable only from butter, coconuts, goats' milk, tomatoes and potatoes. That some of these are rather poor in chlorine does not matter very much. We obtain all the chlorine we need from common salt, either naturally present in food (parsley, for example, contains quite a lot of natural saltiness), or added to it, as in bacon and kippers, or just sprinkled over it. A quick shake from the salt cellar will do far more for 'essential chlorine' than any amount of butter, coconuts, and so on.

Still more of the items, in fact most of them, seem to have originated in Dr Hay's powerful imagination. We are told that mushrooms are a good source of calcium—they contain very little. Coconut is recommended as a source of sulphur—it contains less than most other nuts, and these are not good sources of the element. This nonsense would not matter in most cases, as hardly anyone is deficient in any of the elements on the list, but one or two of the recommendations are definitely dangerous nonsense.

Iron, for example, is essential for the formation of red blood cells, and shortages of it cause anaemia, particularly among pregnant and nursing women. Iron deficiency is unfortunately still quite common, so much so that in Britain iron compounds are added in small quantities to standard bread flour—to a chorus of condemnation from the food reformers, of course, who are opposed to any 'tampering' with food.

Hay dieters, who would of course reject the over-processed, additive-filled modern loaf, would have to rely on his list of iron sources—brazil nuts, figs, egg yolk, rye, pears and oranges. Unfortunately, with the exception of egg yolk, all these foods are *unusually deficient* in iron, and a diet of them not supplemented by meat, lentils, soya beans or some other good source of iron could soon lead to dangerous anaemia.

Similarly, in the important case of iodine, the Hay diet recommendations are so inaccurate as to be dangerous. A shortage of iodine causes the thyroid gland in the neck to swell (the thyroid hormone, thyroxine, requires iodine in its composition), and the disfigurement, goitre, used to be common in places where there is insufficient iodine in the water supply. Derbyshire in Britain is one of these areas, and goitre was often called 'Derbyshire neck' up to about 1900.

The simplest way to get enough iodine, if you live in a deficient district, is to use iodized table salt. If you object in general to 'additives' in food you can usually get enough iodine from fish, watercress, and similar food. If we look in Dr Hay's list we find one real source of iodine—kelp, dried seaweed, which may not be easily obtainable—and otherwise carrots, melons, mushrooms, leeks, and beetroot, possibly the worst sources of iodine that could have been chosen.

The other facet of the Hay Diet, apart from this imaginative treatment of essential elements, was the Ritual. Dr Hay had a fascinating ritual which made his system well known all over the world because it was so easily recognizable. He decided that the various types of food—starches, proteins, fats, and so on—should not be eaten together, but confined to separate meals. 'Starches and sugars require alkaline conditions for complete digestion without fermentation . . . proteins require acid conditions' (*Health Via Food*, 1934) —as a later development, he decided that acid fruits must not be eaten with starches and sugars.

Much the same thought had occurred to Galen, although the basis for this is now lost in antiquity; in the *Governayle of Helthe* we are told: 'Furthermore as Galyen sayeth that at one mele men sholden not ete dyverse metes and therfore at morow [*morning*] ete but bred alone, and at evyn fleshe alone, for when two dyverse metes ben taken at one mele of hem comyn two evyles.'

The 'two evyles' as described in the *Governayle* depended on the fact that in any mixed meal, some of the food must be easily digestible ('lyghte and subtyl mete'), and some more difficult to digest ('grete mete'). The theory was that if you ate the 'lyghte mete' first it would be digested quickly and somehow drag the 'grete mete' through the digestive system too quickly for it to be absorbed properly. If, on the other hand, the less digestible food were eaten first, it would remain in the stomach a long time, preventing the 'lyghte mete' from getting its fair share of attention, and eventually the more digestible food would ferment or rot—'the lyghte mete weryth corupte'.

This theory has a great many resemblances to that of Dr Hay, although nothing in his books suggests that he had ever read Galen or any of the later commentators such as the author of the *Governayle*. Both theories are of equal value—which is to say fascinating as science fiction but completely divorced from the facts.

Even so, the Hay Diet gave an interesting new perspective to the planning of menus. You could have bread, or cheese, but not bread and cheese; meat, or pastry, but not meat pies; cauliflower cheese but not spaghetti cheese; rhubarb, or sugar, but not sweetened rhubarb. Followed to its logical conclusion, the diet should have forbidden the consumption of foods like beans and peas that contain starch and protein together, but apparently the good doctor did not think of that.

Still, as it was, it gave infinite pleasure to the lovers of food ritual and food sacrifice, because there were so many little facets of the theory that could be developed. How much carbo-hydrate had a vegetable to contain, for instance, before it was banished from association with proteins? Was it a mortal sin to dust your lentil croquettes with breadcrumbs, especially if they had been bound together with egg? Was wholemeal bread, which contains protein, and also starch, more or less dangerous than the white bread which was condemned by almost every other food reformer?

Dr Hay seems to have been rather confused himself about this last problem. In one passage of *Health Via Food* he puts the conventional 'natural food' view: 'Nature placed them [vital chemical salts] there for our use in the whole grain, but Man has refined them away, under the impression that he can improve on Nature, or make them more beautiful, or more easily baked, or more easily handled, or stored, or even digested.' However, a little later on in the same book he has obviously thought about the problem of protein and starch co-existing in the loaf, and suddenly utters an anathema against bread of all kinds:

> when we realise the extent to which bread is eaten, the blind dependence placed on this supposed 'staff of life' by almost the entire world, it is not strange that there is so much fermentation and consequent acid formation in the average digestive tract . . . We have seen children scolded, threatened, or even sent from the table because they were unwilling to eat more bread, or to eat it with every other article of food on the table, under the parental misunderstanding of the old idea that 'bread is the staff of life'.

One is reminded of the Fathers of the Church syllogizing their way round some particularly awkward disagreement between Aristotle and St Paul, except that Dr Hay was no Aquinas.

One side-effect of the popularity of the diet was a whole new industry in writing cookery books for those trying to conform to the system and still make any sort of appetizing meal—people like the 'fanatical Hay-dieter' in a 1936 *Punch* cartoon who terrifies other diners in a restaurant with the cry, 'I've been watching you, sir. You're courting disaster. Good Heavens! Mixing carbo-hydrates with proteins'. Dr Hay's collaborator Doris Grant was an enthusiastic compiler of such cookery books, and even produced one for Hay-dieters in wartime—*Feeding the Family in Wartime—based on the new knowledge of nutrition*, which must have made one more difficulty for the ration-bound community.

It may have seemed unnecessary to dissect the theories of the unfortunate Dr Hay so minutely—after all, he died long ago. Sad to say, however, his soul, and his pernicious ideas about nutrition, go marching on to this day, still appearing in the pages of diet and health magazines. Sometimes the theories are credited to him, but often they are presented as if they are the latest fruits of deep nutritional research.

For example, in a book published in 1956, we find, with a sense of *déjà vu*, that the body requires sixteen elements for its nourishment—Oxygen, Hydrogen, Carbon, Nitrogen and so on, and that Oxygen can be obtained from mint, parsley, rhubarb, tomatoes, onions, potatoes and horseradish. This list is longer by three items than Dr Hay's original, and I suspect that the author may be representative of a wild new generation of Hay-worshippers who are prepared to tamper with the holy writ of *Health Via Food*. However, on combinations of foods, ortho-doxy prevails—starches, fats and sugars must not be eaten at the same meal as proteins or acid fruits.

Even later, in 1962, E. Gilbert Oakley published *Better Health from Health Foods and Herbs* (Max Parrish), with the same list of the sixteen essential elements, and the correct combinations of types of food. Mr Oakley is a professed disciple of Dr Hay, so it is not surprising to find him following the Hay diet so closely. However, as Hay had little to say about vitamins in his books, this gives Mr Oakley a chance to strike out on his own—which he does, in great style.

Having taken to his heart the technique of converting vegetables to liquid in 'juicers', he proposes proudly:

Look for these vital vitamins in the fruit and vegetables you *drink*.

Raspberry	A B B_2 C	Grape	C A B_2 B
Strawberry	A B B_2 E	Banana	Nil
Watercress	A B B_2 C E	Blackberry	C
Carrot	B_1 B_2 C	Turnip	A C
Orange	C	Parsley	A
Pear	B B_1 B_2 C	Radish	A B B_2 C
Pineapple	B E	Spinach	A
Peach	A B B_2 C	Celery	A B B_2 C

I quote this table at length because it illustrates so well the air of certainty and scientific accuracy which pervades so much of modern health food literature. The names of the vitamins are real (although one might wonder what exactly is meant by 'vitamin B' as distinct from B_1 or the B_2 complex), and the writer was editor of a well known and widely read magazine on health matters. Tables of the vitamin contents of fruit, vege-tables, and other foodstuffs are readily available. So the reader would assume, taking all these factors into account, that the table above was substantially accurate.

In fact, it would be just about as accurate if Mr Oakley had put the names of the vitamins into a hat and drawn them out blindfold. You could 'look for' vitamin A, as invited, in grapes, turnips, radishes and celery, but you would not find any. On the other hand, carrots, which are not credited with vitamin A at all, actually contain more than almost any other vegetable or fruit. Strawberries, with a higher vitamin C content than any other fruit except blackcurrants do not rate a mention for this, while pears, grapes, and celery, extremely low in this vitamin, are recommended as sources. Oranges, richer in vitamin B_1 than most other fruit, are ignored, while carrots, rather poor in this vitamin, are promoted. And the poor banana, really quite good as a source of A, B_1 and B_2, and not too short of C, is condemned as useless.

In fact, between pages 27 and 66 of his book, Mr Oakley seems to have had a change of heart (or a change of hat to pick the vitamins out of), and on the later page recommends bananas for vitamin A and oranges for vitamin B. However, this later table seems to be just as arbitrary as the earlier one.

It is a constant complaint in magazines such as Mr Oakley's *Here's Health* and its modern successors that the great pioneers of medical and dietetic reform are always derided and obstructed by the orthodox medical profession. This is, unfortunately, often true, and I have tried in this book to set matters more in perspective. However, the sort of nonsense I have quoted above does more harm to the cause of food reform than a dozen hostile medical Establishments. To develop and test new theories of nutrition is a useful and praiseworthy task, but to support them by misstatements of fact that could be detected by a schoolchild is merely stupid.

Perhaps the most happily ungoverned book of this kind in recent years has been *Natural Remedies for Common Ailments* by Constance Mellor (C. W. Daniel, London, 1973). The book is extremely entertaining and, of course, opposed to modern methods of food production:

Manufactured foodstuffs are mass-produced in factories and laboratories. They are, for the most part, foodless foods, of value only to the producers, who make big profits out of them. They are tinned, bottled, packeted rubbish, useless as proper nourishment for the body. Foods that are tampered by Man—i.e. heat-treated, processed, tinned, bottled or preserved—are killed stone-dead by the tampering, and certain it is that dead foods cannot put life into our bodies.

Salt is another enemy to well-being, and, according to Ms Mellor, even a source of cancer:

A grave dietetic error is the eating of too much salt . . . It can so easily be taken in excess because so many of the foods we eat are already salted, to preserve them. For example, factory-made butter contains about 8 teaspoonfuls of salt to the pound ($\frac{1}{2}$ a teaspoonful to the ounce). Bakers use salt heavily in breadmaking. Tinned meats etc. contain salt; so do sausages, bacon, cheese, gravy flavourings, ice-cream and aspirin tablets.

It is not quite clear why aspirin tablets get into this list of foodstuffs at all, so the fact that they contain no salt is probably irrelevant. However, the only actual figures quoted, those for butter, suggest a salt content of about 5 per cent, which happens to be five times higher than the most heavily-salted butter on the market, so the reader is left wondering where Ms Mellor found her 'facts'.

Her strong objection to salt in diet arose from her belief that it caused cancer. She describes a complicated process by which the salt is broken down in the body to chlorine and caustic soda, and how the latter, a strong irritant, stimulates cells to multiply and form 'tumourous growths'. How the body manages to make the caustic soda is not explained—many industrial chemists would be delighted if such a simple reaction could be achieved even in a chemical plant.

Quite often in this book, as in so many other diet reform treatises, you get the impression that 'chemicals' and 'drugs' are harmful if used by the wicked food manufacturers, or prescribed by orthodox doctors, but undergo a miraculous transformation if recommended by naturopaths. For example, monosodium glutamate (see pp 69–70), a popular additive to savoury foods, is condemned roundly by Ms Mellor and most other natural food enthusiasts as a harmful 'chemical' foisted on the public. Yet she goes on to recommend glutamic acid hydrochloride as a natural way of preventing anaemia. Monosodium glutamate is immediately converted to glutamic acid hydrochloride when it reaches the stomach.

Similarly, while she condemns the addition of nitrates to foods such as bacon and ham (they are used in the curing salts), we read: 'Dr Paul Kirsch has . . . written a very helpful book called *The Curability of Cancer* (British Biochemic Association). He too believes that cancer can be caused by a shortage of potassium; this can be remedied by daily doses of specially-prepared potassium nitrate.' So potassium nitrate used by the bacon-curer is poison, potassium nitrate prepared by Dr Kirsch is a cure for cancer.

One way round this difficulty, often adopted by health food writers, is to divide chemicals into 'natural' and 'artificial' types. If a manufacturer uses, say, nitrates, his products are artificial. If a food reformer uses nitrates, they are natural. This sort of double-think is illustrated very well in a passage from Sir Albert Howard, writing about fertilizers (quoted in *A Complete Guide to Vitamins*, J. I. Rodale, Rodale Press, 1968):

> . . . natural nitrate has something that the artificial lacks . . . Chilean nitrate contains small amounts of vital impurities such as magnesium, iodine, boron, calcium, potassium, lithium and strontium, which are to plants what the vitamins in fresh foods are to human beings. It has been found that natural nitrate does something that makes apples stay on trees; that it does something to corn that results in better live stock fattened on it; that chickens raised on nitrated feed lay better eggs of greater fertility. It is just as impossible to make artificial nitrates that duplicate natural nitrates as it is to make artificial sea water that contains all the elements of natural sea water.

Here is an example of the enormous magnetism exercised by the word 'natural'. Mr Rodale, in whose book this passage is quoted, is a writer normally passionately dedicated to the use of organic manures, and as passionately opposed to 'chemicals' in agriculture. Sodium nitrate, whether the impure form from Chile or an entirely artificial type, is the last thing he would normally recommend as plant food (and, in fact, the passage is quoted in a chapter headed 'Unavoidable Nitrates Destroy Vitamin A', and concerned in general to condemn the use of nitrates in agriculture or food). But the fact that Sir Albert is able to distinguish his nitrate as 'natural' casts such a charm that we are left with the impression that nitrates are wonderful —as long as they are not pure.

8 Magic Potions

Ever since the alchemists started their search for the Elixir of Life, the great remedy that would enable the discoverer of the Philosophers' Stone to enjoy his riches for an indefinite number of years, people have been trying to convince themselves or others that there are magic constituents in some foods that can miraculously prolong life, eliminate disease, and roll back the years to an imagined flower of youth when we could all display bodies like Greek gods or goddesses, clear eyes, perfect skin, and unquenchable stamina.

The older elixirs tended to be described as extracts from exotic plants or animals, usually employed by hitherto unknown tribes of virile Methuselahs, and only just discovered for the benefit of the etiolated inhabitants of Europe or America. When so much of the world was unknown, and the maps contained great blank spaces where no white man had penetrated, it was easy to believe such tales, and the reputed unicorns' horns or snake oils were accepted as genuine products of exploration.

The same sales story has not lost its power even in modern times, if one judges by the success of the sale of ginseng in Europe and the USA. Ginseng is a mildly stimulant plant which might have been more exciting if tea and coffee had not already reached Europe, but because it comes from Korea and is used in China, two countries possibly less familiar to Westerners than any others, it arrived in the West with a reputation for rejuvenation and the restoration of sexual powers.

'Korean ginseng has been reverently used in the Orient for thousands of years, and is reputed by the Chinese to be of great value in preserving strength, vigour, and vitality. They also call it the rejuvenation herb, and its enthusiasts consider it the panacea of all diseases,' says one advertising leaflet, while another points out that it 'has been reputed for many thousands of years to improve the function of the brain and memory as well as restoring vitality and virility'. One wonders why the Chinese, a sensible and economical race, are wasting so much money on training doctors.

In the nineteenth and early twentieth centuries, the unknown geographical world was shrinking fast, but there was a new and wonderful source of mysterious remedies for every ill in the world of chemistry and physics. The fashion grew for wonder-foods to contain new elements, or to give off mysterious rays, or in some other way to have originated in the latter-day alchemists' laboratories. The march of science was then still triumphal and beneficient, without its modern sinister side, and no cure-all was complete without its collection of long incomprehensible words on the label—such as the *glycerophosphates* which were supposed to rebuild the shattered brain and nervous system of the tired Victorian businessman, and can still be found among the ingredients of modern 'tonic' wines.

The modern writer on fringe diet matters has to steer a careful course between the two extremes. His readers want to hear a certain amount of nutritional jargon, and will not be satisfied unless the new discovery has its share of vitamins (preferably one or two vitamins hitherto unknown to orthodox nutritional science), enzymes, minerals and trace elements, essential fatty acids and amino-acids, and so on, but there must be no suggestion that it contains 'chemicals'. If possible there should be a fraction of a per cent that is 'completely unanalysable' and can therefore be supposed to contain the key to the wonderful effects. Primitive methods of production and a history of use among the unspoiled peasants of Anatolia are, however, still potent selling points, and if the product can be prepared only by hand-grinding in a quern, so much the better. It often seems that to attract the modern health-food enthusiast the manufacturer should invert the old hygienic slogan and make sure that his product is touched by as many human hands as possible.

Bread   As has emerged several times in previous chapters, it seems that there is no food product which inspires such emotion as bread, and the choice of wholemeal or white carries the same overtones of religious intolerance as would the choice of pork or beef in various parts of the Indian continent.

A typical description of white bread, taken from a health magazine, runs as follows: 'White bread is anything but the staff of life; it is a denatured, devitalized creation that is totally unfit for human food; a substance that causes a clogging of the system, possessing hardly any nutritional value . . .' Criticisms of white bread in similar terms are common in all diet reform literature: another magazine shows pictures of slices of wholemeal, brown, and white bread, with the caption that this shows the transformation of bread from 'food' to 'toxin'.

This sort of exaggeration is, in the end, self-defeating: very few people would deny that wholemeal bread is a nutritious and pleasant food, though rather heavy if you have to eat a lot of it for economic reasons, and that it contains rather more vitamins, trace elements, and fibre than white bread. But to claim that white bread is 'unfit for human food' is sheer arrogance.

As explained in Chapter 3, white flour is made by crushing the wheat grain between rollers, and then sieving out the bran. Unfortunately the wheatgerm is sieved out as well, as the rollers spread it out into a flat disc that cannot pass the mesh of the sieve. The flour that results is classified by the percentage of the total meal that is retained in the flour—100 per cent extraction is wholemeal flour, with the germ and the bran from the outside of the grain, 85 per cent extraction gave the rather grey flour that went into the wartime British loaf, and 70 per cent extraction gives the modern white loaf. Not only is the colour paler, but the 70 per cent extraction flour makes a lighter and more open loaf.

If it were left in this state, the white loaf would have, compared with wholewheat, less protein and fat, about half the calcium and iron, about three-quarters of the thiamin (vitamin B_1), one-third of the nicotinic acid and one-quarter of the riboflavin (both B_2 vitamins). However, in nearly every bread-eating country except France and Holland the flour is enriched by adding thiamin, nicotinic acid, riboflavin, iron and calcium to bring the nutritional levels up to or above the level in wholemeal flour. Riboflavin is not added in Britain, although it is used in many other countries. The amount of calcium available to the body from white bread may in fact be greater than that from wholemeal bread, as bran contains a material called *phytic acid* that combines with calcium to make a non-digestible compound. The other components, starch and so on, are about the same for all types of flour, and the important vitamins A, C, and D are not present to any great extent in bread.

It may seem odd to mill out certain nutrients and then have to put them back, but this process makes it easier to eliminate much of the bran that tends to make loaves heavy. The bran is of course useful, if you happen to like wholemeal bread, because it stimulates the bowels to regular action. Dr D. P. Burkitt of the British Medical Research Council has pointed out (1975) that a number of abdominal complaints such as appendicitis, hiatus hernia, and haemorrhoids, and even vari-cose veins, may be due to a lack of sufficient movement, and points out that rural Africans, who eat very coarse whole-grain foods, rarely suffer from such diseases except when they adopt a 'Western' type of diet.

This can hardly be considered a revelation: Sir Henry Thompson, a great nutritional expert, wrote in his book *Food and Feeding* (1891):

I have just adverted to the bread of the labourer, and recom-mended that it should be made from entire wholemeal; but it should not be too coarsely ground . . . At the same time, no portion of the husk of the grain should be removed from the wheat when ground, whether coarsely or finely, into meal. That a partial removal is systematically advocated by some as an improvement, is one of the numerous illustrations of the modern and almost universal craze which just now exists among food purveyors of almost every description for eliminating all inert or innutritious material from the food we eat. This extraordinary care to employ nothing in our diet but matter which has nutritive value, that is, that can be absorbed into the system, is founded upon want of elementary knowledge of the first principles of nutrition.

On the other hand, Sir Henry was too sensible to insist that bran was the only way to introduce fibre into the system. He recommended wholemeal bread for the 'labourer' because at the time the working-man's diet would have included a lot of bread and very few vegetables, but I think he would have been amused or appalled to see people who can easily afford the most varied diet solemnly swallowing bran as the panacea for all ills. If you like wholemeal bread, it is a good way of getting the fibre you need: if not, you can easily obtain the same fibrous material from vegetables such as cabbage, carrots, swedes (rutabaga), beetroot, and so on, and you will also get a useful supply of vitamins and minerals from the vegetables. It is not generally realized, for example, that swedes even after cooking contain more vitamin C than many fresh fruits.

Yogurt   Milk soured by the bacterium *Lactobacillus bulgaricus* has been popular for centuries in the Balkans, where it is very difficult to keep milk sweet, and similar preparations are made all over the Middle East, the Black Sea coast, and in the southern areas of Russia. Many of these products are made from mares' milk, a reminder that they originated with the wandering Tartar hordes.

Several medical writers in the nineteenth century pointed out how stable yogurt and the other soured milk products were compared with meat: the lactic acid produced by the bacteria is a powerful preservative, and is in fact the main reason why pickles and sauerkraut can be kept for long periods. A vogue started for taking such milk products as a kind of preservative for the digestive system, with the idea that the bacteria might be introduced permanently into the human intestine: an Italian doctor called Rovighi wrote an enthusiastic paper in 1892 on the benefits of *kephir*, a Caucasian alcoholic drink made by fermenting the milk of mares, goats, or ewes. He drank a litre and a half of this every day, and claimed that it prevented 'auto-intoxication' (a phrase popular at the time, and having nothing to do with the considerable alcohol content of kephir, but derived from the idea that dangerous bacteria could breed in the large intestine unless some agency such as lactic acid was present to stop them).

The craze might have died away, had it not come to the notice of Ilya Metchnikoff, possibly the greatest biologist of his time after Pasteur, with whom he worked for some years, and winner of the Nobel Prize for Medicine for his work on the functions of the white blood corpuscles in combating bacteria. Metchnikoff, in the true optimistic mood of his time, had already decided that the elimination of most disease was only a matter of time and the application of the methods laid down by Pasteur and himself, and set out to find out what made people grow old and die in the absence of any specific disease. He decided that this was due to the presence of the intestinal bacteria, and that lactic acid, in the form of sour milk products, would therefore hold up the process of ageing.

He was greatly encouraged in his theory by the discovery that various Bulgarian tribes, whose diet regularly included yogurt, were believed to produce large numbers of people of great longevity, and as yogurt was less alcoholic than kephir Metchnikoff recommended it warmly in his book *The Prolongation of Life*, which had a wide circulation in the early years of the twentieth century. How tribes with no written records were able to keep a tally on their oldest inhabitants was never explained, but no one seemed to bother about this (or indeed about the tribes) after they had served their purposes as an inspiration to sour-milk drinkers. Yogurt itself, kephir, *koumiss* (another Tartar preparation from mares' milk), and *leben*, a North African preparation from cows', goats' or buffalos' milk, became the latest diet fad. Yogurt has had a revival in recent years as a useful outlet for skimmed milk that would otherwise have to be used for animal food, and British consumption alone is over 260 million cartons per year. Gayelord Hauser, doyen of the American diet reformers, was an enthusiast for yogurt and counted it as one of his 'Wonder Foods', thus introducing it to many dieters.

However, despite its reputation, yogurt can hardly be considered a wonder food. Metchnikoff was a brilliant biologist, but this did not prevent him from being wrong sometimes, and no work since his time has produced any evidence that lactic acid or the 'acidophilous milks' (as yogurt, kephir, koumiss and so on are collectively called) have much effect on health, let alone longevity. Many writers still quote the number of centenarians among the Bulgars as a testimonial for yogurt, but if one accepts this argument there is the rather inconvenient evidence of even longer-lived tribes in Peru whose main diet consists of guinea pigs.

It is better to accept that yogurt is a useful but dull item of food, with the same protein and minerals as the skimmed milk from which it is made, almost all the same vitamins (although vitamins A, C, and D tend to disappear during the commercial production), and, in the commercial product, less fat, which may suit some slimmers. Home-made yogurt, produced from full-cream milk, has almost exactly the same food value as the milk, and if you prefer to be able to eat your milk with a spoon rather than drinking it, yogurt may be useful.

It is an ironic fact that those writers on diet who make the greatest claims for yogurt and still quote Metchnikoff's original praise for it are also those who tend to recommend wholefoods and the use of fresh, uncooked, unprocessed products in diet. One can only suppose that they have never read Metchnikoff at first hand, because an essential part of his theory was that bacteria in food must be destroyed by thorough cooking: 'Obviously we should eat no raw food, but confine our diet rigidly to food that has been thoroughly cooked or sterilised. The exclusion of "wild" microbes and the introduction of beneficial microbes, such as those of lactic acid fermentation, must be of great service to health.' (*The Nature of Man*, 1903) *Sweeteners*   One of the few points of agreement among the many conflicting schools of food reform is that white sugar is bad for us. 'Refined' becomes a distinctly pejorative word in the literature, although curiously enough 'pure' is all right— 'pure food' is the nutritious stuff sold in health food stores, while 'refined food' is the deleterious, devitalized, denatured brew forced upon us by the wicked food manufacturers—or so one would believe after a short course of food reform literature.

On the other hand, even a cursory examination of the same literature will show that the popular 'health' diets tend to include molasses, honey, brown sugar of various kinds, carob bean, maple syrup, dried fruit, and a lot of other very sweet things, which are often claimed to be essential articles of diet, with qualities only previously paralleled by nectar or Amrita for securing long life and radiant health. It cannot therefore be that mere sweetness has offended the puritan susceptibilities of the diet writers.

The cold fact is that in the West we nearly all eat too much sugar, of all kinds, and it does not matter very much what kind of sugar it is. White sugar is pure sucrose, whether it is derived from sugar-cane or beet, and possibly the purest foodstuff available, in that it consists of sucrose only, with barely a fraction of a per cent of impurity. Sucrose is made up of two simpler sugars linked together, glucose, sometimes called dextrose or grape sugar, and fructose, occasionally called laevulose or fruit sugar, and within a very short time of sucrose being eaten in any form, it is converted in the body to these two simpler materials. Glucose is one of the most important sources of energy, or calories, requiring insulin to complete its digestion (diabetics lack enough natural insulin to manage this). Fructose is also converted to energy, but by a different mechanism. If we eat more sugar than we need for our normal energy requirements, the spare glucose is converted first to glycogen, a kind of starch, and then to fat, so that habitual overeating of sugar makes us overweight, and some doctors would say liable to heart disease and a number of other serious illnesses.

So how are the 'dietetic' sweet foods different? The answer is that they are not. Maple syrup is made of sucrose, and therefore no different in nutritional value or danger to an equal amount of white sugar and water. It tastes different, because of traces of other materials, and many people (myself included) like the taste. But if we eat too much food sweetened with maple syrup, we will suffer exactly the same ills as if we ate too much refined white sugar.

Of the 'brown' sugars, one of the most common is the large-crystal Demerara sugar, often served by food reformers with an air of conscious superiority over the unfortunate herd who are still poisoning themselves with white sugar. Demerara sugar is, in fact, refined white sugar that has been coloured with a very small trace of burnt sugar (caramel) or molasses. Many people prefer it in coffee because of the faint treacly taste of the additive, and it can be obtained in large misshapen chips that dissolve very slowly, so that your cup of coffee tastes sweeter at the end than at the beginning. However, pleasant though it is, Demerara sugar is no more 'natural' than a stick of seaside rock.

The various grades of 'soft' brown sugar (Barbados, soft black, 'pieces', and so on) are products of sugar refining taken out of the process before all the molasses has been removed. Again, they taste pleasant in puddings and so forth, but consist almost entirely of sucrose and have the same nutritional values and disadvantages.

Molasses or black treacle is the syrup left over from sugar-cane when solid sugar has been removed. It has been a favourite magic ingredient in the food reform kitchen for many years, and one would imagine from the literature that it contained some mysterious essence so far removed from the sucrose of white sugar that they had nothing in common. In fact, apart from about 27 per cent water, molasses contains about 47 per cent of sucrose and 20 per cent of glucose, the normal product of sucrose digestion. So if your diet is over-burdened with sugar, changing over from white sugar to molasses will not help you much—in fact, as molasses is a lot less sweet than white sugar, you will probably have to use more of it to flavour your food, thus taking in as much sugar as before, or perhaps even more.

Molasses also contains a residue of mineral salts from the sugar-cane (and the processing machinery), and could provide you with iron and calcium if these were not available in the rest of your diet. On the other hand, you could get these minerals from vegetables just as easily, without the accompanying large dose of sugar. Molasses also has a small amount of protein (about half that contained in the same quantity of milk), but no vitamins worth considering. If by some Robinson Crusoe chance you found yourself having to live on either pure white sugar or molasses, and no other food, you would be marginally better off with the molasses. However, as you would die from deficiency diseases quite soon in either case, the advantages are not great. Under normal circumstances there is no reason to eat molasses rather than any other form of sugar unless you actually prefer it.

Honey has been the subject of more romantic and magical nonsense during the last few years than almost any other article of diet, and, as with molasses, the writers on health foods tend to give the impression that honey contains large amounts of nutrients which are unique and unobtainable from other food. In fact, three-quarters of honey is made up from glucose, fructose, and sucrose, in exactly the same proportions as if you took ordinary white sugar and boiled it with water, or simply digested it. Another 20 per cent is moisture, and the remaining 5 per cent contains a very small amount of protein, beeswax that has not been separated from the honey, traces of acids, and a small amount of mineral material. The vitamin content of honey is almost negligible.

So, apart from the taste, honey has the same food value as a rather smaller amount of ordinary sugar—a pound of honey is roughly equivalent to 12oz of sugar. Most of the literature about honey, apart from the sheer magic phrases like 'it contains a small residue which is entirely unanalysable'—which is true of any material if you make the 'small residue' small enough—are claims that it is preservative, that it kills germs, that it soothes wounds, and so on. These sound impressive until one reflects that sugar has exactly the same preservative effects, as any jam-maker knows, and in fact the argument is exactly the same as that used by Frederick Slare in the eighteenth century to prove that sugar was a valuable health food (see page 32). Claims that honey produces energy are of course true, but again so would a dose of sugar in any form, white, brown, glucose or molasses. And as honey contains hardly anything else except sugar and water, it can just as easily be overeaten as white sugar.

Carob beans have become something of a craze, as their extract is very sweet, like maple syrup, and can be made into confectionery similar to boiled sugar products like fudge or toffee. Various advertisements have appeared in health food magazines and stores for candy bars made of carob, usually carrying the claim that these 'are the healthy way to indulge a sweet tooth', or similar implications.

The carob-tree, algarroba, or locust-tree (*Ceratonia siliqua*), has been known for centuries in the Mediterranean area. In Sicily the sweet pods are often fermented to make a local liqueur, and the syrup has been used as a honey-substitute in Italy, Greece, and the Near East. In many places the pods are given whole to animals as a fodder supplement.

There is nothing mysterious about the sweetness: carob syrup contains large proportions of glucose, fructose, and sucrose, and is in fact very similar to honey in its composition. Sweet-meats made of carob therefore have almost exactly the same components as ordinary toffees or any other confection made by boiling cane-sugar, as boiling converts some of the sucrose in ordinary sugar to a mixture of glucose and fructose. Carob candy bars will therefore also have exactly the same effects on the teeth and the digestion as sweets made from cane-sugar.

One amusing aspect of the advertising of carob candy bars, which illustrates the desperate attempts to enlist almost any selling point that can be raised, is the suggestion in some advertisements that the carob-bean was used by John the Baptist during his time in the wilderness ('And the same John had his raiment of camel's hair, and a leathern girdle about his loins; and his meat was locusts and wild honey.' Matthew 3, 4). This depends on the illiterate notion that his food was the locust-bean and not the insect, although there is no real doubt in the original text. Owing to a curious gap in the Jewish hygienic laws, as set out in the Book of Leviticus, locusts and grasshoppers generally are not unclean animals, and John was being perfectly orthodox in eating them. Many African peoples still eat locusts, which have an appreciable food value. It was as well for St John that he ate the insect and not the bean,

otherwise his diet would have consisted almost entirely of sugar.
Mineral supplements   One of the most popular, and profitable aspects of 'magic ingredient' dietetics is the recommendation and supply of minerals which are supposed to be needed
by the body but lacking in modern diet. From the journalists'
point of view the subject is popular because there is an almost
unlimited list of mineral elements that actually exist in the body,
albeit in tiny traces, so that after the obvious ones like iron and
calcium have been written to death, there are copper, zinc,
chromium, cobalt, and so on ready to furnish fresh articles.
Each one can be credited with an essential role in the metabolism, either from textbooks or from the inspiration of the
moment, and a few phrases composed to show how modern
processing removes all the valuable ingredient from food.

From the manufacturers' point of view, minerals are even
better. The amounts needed of even the most important ones
are relatively tiny, so a small tablet or a spoonful of elixir can
really provide all the copper, zinc, etc. needed by the average
person, and, most important, the compounds themselves are
nearly all extremely cheap.

As an example of 'mineral supplement' thinking (and also an
example of the tremendous powers of double-think possessed
by writers on health foods), take two articles in the same issue
of a health magazine. One, castigating the producers of white
bread for their deplorable product, says: 'Moreover we have
to face the frightening fact that the average loaf of bread contains a large quantity of crude calcium added by the bakers,
and this causes hardening of the arteries and ages the system.'
A few pages on, in 'Dolomite—the Stone that Protects Your
Heart' we find: 'A shortage of calcium must inevitably result
in a weakened heartbeat which . . . cannot be strengthened as
long as the calcium is deficient.'

In some magazines this anomaly would be explained simply
on the basis that 'crude calcium' was no substitute for calcium
in living plants, or some similar 'organic' explanation, but in
this case the magic ingredient which is effectively being sold to
the reader is powdered dolomite, a kind of limestone which is
best obtained by scraping pieces off the outsides of large

buildings, as dolomite is a popular building stone. A 'cruder' form of calcium could scarcely be imagined.

However, as has been said, writers on health diets seem to possess an infinite capacity for 'double-think'—the ability to believe two mutually contradictory things at the same time—and when it comes to finding 'facts' to support their theories, we enter a field of intellectual endeavour that can only be termed *free-range thinking*, not confined by any slavish respect for fact or even consistency. Take, for example, this description from a leaflet on Dr Schuessler's *Biochemic Tissue-Salts*, some of the most widely-distributed mineral supplements on the market:

> *Nat. mur.* is the *water-distributing* tissue-salt. It enters into the composition of every fluid and solid of the body. Because of its powerful affinity for water, it controls the ebb and flow of bodily fluids; its prime function being to maintain the proper degree of moisture throughout the system. Without this tissue-salt, cell division and normal growth could not proceed.

Imagine that, having read this, the anxious customer rushes off to the local health food store to get hold of some *Nat. mur.* before normal growth ceases altogether. He finds it among the other Tissue-Salts as a small bottle of tiny tablets.

And what is in the tablets? Milk sugar plus a very small amount of the magical *Nat. mur.*, which is sodium chloride, common salt. The customer might have a sneaking suspicion that there are cheaper ways of buying salt, supposing that he or she is actually short of this mineral, but, just in case there is something really special about the Tissue-Salts, consults some of the books on diet displayed alongside Dr Schuessler's little miracles. Open at random, and here is a chapter entitled *Salt is a Poison!*, which shows conclusively that not only salt added at table, but salt put into foods by the manufacturers, is rapidly causing 'impairment of the stomach'. Salt is apparently a 'vile adulteration' of natural food.

At last, if he has not slipped away in complete bewilderment, the customer will understand the fundamental truth about health foods—minerals bought at great expense through the health food store are valuable diet supplements, minerals added by food manufacturers are dangerous chemicals. It does not matter that sometimes the minerals are the same in both cases.

For instance, two of the other Biochemic Tissue-Salts are *Calc. sulph.* and *Silica. Calc. sulph.* is better known as Plaster of Paris, and used to be added to cake flour by really un-scrupulous bakers to make their fruit cakes stay up better without eggs. *Silica* is sand, and one would have to go back into the pages of history to find out when this was last used to adulterate sugar and similar food. But if Dr Schuessler has put his seal of approval on them, plaster and sand become valuable diet supplements.

In fact, the chances of anyone in the developed Western countries being short of any of the minerals necessary for life is very remote, except for iron, iodine, and fluorine in certain circumstances. Iron is the most serious shortage, and many people may be getting rather less than they need to maintain the proper level of red blood corpuscles. Mineral supplements are one answer, and are normally given to pregnant and nursing mothers and people who have recently had serious operations, but for the average person it would be simpler and more pleasant to increase the amount of iron in food. Meat such as lamb's liver is very rich in iron, but for those who do not wish to eat meat there is plenty of the mineral in eggs, beans, dried fruit and nuts (including peanut butter).

Iodine may be lacking in people a long way from the sea, especially if their water is very pure and soft (see page 93). Iodized table salt is the easiest way to get enough iodine if you live in such an area, or you can eat more seafood or water-cress and other water-plants, which accumulate iodine.

Fluorine is necessary for healthy teeth, as it acts as a harden-ing agent for the apatite in tooth enamel that forms the wearing surfaces. Fluorine is present naturally as fluoride in many sources of water, and people in these areas do not have to worry about their source of the mineral, as not only do they absorb it with water, but the local plants accumulate it. Where fluorine is lacking, the simplest solution is for the public authorities to add fluoride to the water supply. Unfortunately this step has been hysterically opposed in some areas by groups of people who seem determined to sacrifice the teeth of their neighbours' children so that they themselves can feel virtuous about ensuring an 'uncontaminated' water supply, forgetting that it is only because of the unnatural processes of filtration and chlorination that they are saved from the natural joys of typhoid and cholera. I do not know whether any of these groups have yet suggested that they should be supplied with *absolutely* untreated water, but if they were, we should soon hear less of them.

Vitamin supplements   Since the discovery of the various vitamins during the earlier years of this century, they have inevitably caught the public attention, and a great deal of folklore has gathered around them, sedulously fostered by those whose business it is to sell vitamin pills, 'tonics', special foodstuffs, or diet systems.

Typical remarks and beliefs are, for example, that cooking destroys nearly all the vitamins in food, or that canned/frozen/dried foods are completely devoid of them. I have a fairly modern book, by a doctor, on my shelf that says categorically that *all* the vitamins in food are destroyed within a few minutes of just cutting it up or shredding it, and that therefore we must eat all our food not only raw but literally whole. Compost or 'organically' grown vegetables are believed to contain vitamins that commercially-grown food has not, and, inevitably, over all the stories is the suggestion that we can only be really healthy and happy if we increase our vitamin intake by swallowing tablets, capsules, or mysterious fluids called 'health cocktails'. 'Over 40 *everybody* needs G - - - - - - - - every day,' 'If you need quick action vitamins take these,' and so on. Barbara Cartland, rattling about with her ninety vitamin pills a day, is held up as a shining example of modern healthy living!

The facts are that very few people in Western countries are short of any of the vitamins, and when slight deficiencies occur because of peculiarities of diet, they can easily be put right either by changing the diet or by the occasional dose of whichever one vitamin is lacking. Daily medication with these 'blockbuster' treatments is quite unnecessary.

Some vitamins are so widespread in all types of food that the 'deficiency disease' caused by their absence from the diet has never been seen outside the laboratory. Doctors have to give volunteers specially purified diets which have been laboriously denuded of the vitamin, so that they can see what happens without it. Such vitamins are *biotin* and *choline*, in the B_2 group. Choline occurs in almost every food containing protein, meat, fish, eggs, milk, beans and other pulses, etc., and biotin is actually synthesized in the human intestine. It was only discovered because it is inactivated by large amounts of raw egg white, and a health crank who ate sixteen raw eggs a day (and nothing else) developed the beginnings of the deficiency disease. Vitamin E, currently popular as 'the rejuvenation vitamin', is so widely distributed in margarine, cooking and salad oils, and other fats that no one in the West is likely to suffer from a deficiency, although in some parts of the Third World not enough is obtained in the diet.

Some vitamins are actually harmful if taken too enthusiastically. The fat-soluble vitamins A and D, if eaten to excess for the normal requirements of the body, are stored in the liver and may easily build up to poisonous levels. Many babies in the USA have been made acutely ill (vomiting, diarrhoea, loss of weight, and permanent kidney damage) by anxious mothers dosing them with large amounts of cod liver and halibut liver oils, and similar good sources of vitamin D. In Britain in 1974, a health food enthusiast killed himself by vitamin A overdosage: he drank several pints of carrot juice every day, and also took multivitamin pills containing more of the vitamin.

Contrary to the suggestions in health food literature, women's magazines, and similar well-informed sources, most vitamins survive food processing and cooking very well. Vitamin C is the most sensitive to heat, and does not survive drying processes, but the fact that it can cope with a good deal of heat is shown by the surprising evidence that the average British family gets most of its vitamin C from potatoes, boiled, mashed, or even chipped. Several vegetables have such rich stores of the vitamin that they are still valuable sources even after normal cooking: swedes (rutabaga) and turnips, for example, contain more vitamin C after boiling than many raw fresh fruits. Folic acid (folacin) of the B$_2$ group is also sensitive to cooking, and is one of the many good reasons for eating green salads as regularly as possible—lettuce and similar salad vegetables are good sources of the vitamin.

Vitamin B$_1$ (thiamin) is not much affected by boiling, but dry heat, like toasting bread, will destroy it. As it is soluble in water, it tends to be lost if vegetables are boiled in a large excess of water and this is poured away: for better flavour and preserved vitamin B$_1$ vegetables should be boiled in as little water as possible, and any vegetable water left over saved for stock or soups. Riboflavin, of the B$_2$ group, is not much affected by heat, but is destroyed by sunlight, so apart from the risk of souring it, you should try not to leave your milk on the doorstep in the sun, because milk is a primary source of riboflavin.

Processing under modern conditions leaves far more vitamins in food than most diet reformers like to admit. Vitamins A, B$_1$, C, folic acid and pantothenic acid (of the B$_2$ group), are largely destroyed by drying processes, but the vitamin C is often replaced in instant mashed potato because it is recognized that potatoes are traditionally an important source of the vitamin. If you do not keep your mashed potato waiting around too long before serving it, 'instant' gives as much vitamin C as mash from fresh potatoes. Freezing affects very few of the vitamins: pantothenic acid and vitamin E are the only ones seriously diminished.

Slight risks of vitamin deficiencies do, of course, exist in Western countries, but only in rather specialized circumstances. Pregnant and nursing mothers and teenage girls should make sure that their vitamin A intake is kept up with plenty of butter, margarine, eggs, and green vegetables—if the girls are figure-conscious the fats may be taboo, but green salads and plenty of green cooked vegetables should be welcome. Those who dislike all milk products may go short of riboflavin, and should make sure of eating yeast extract, soya beans or flour, nuts, or some other alternative source.

The bedsit girl, who may tend to live on hasty meals from

cans or packets, and probably does not eat potatoes because of her figure, needs regular fresh fruit, either whole or as juice, to keep up the supply of vitamin C. It is an ironic fact that many such girls spend a great deal of money on expensive cosmetics and moisturising creams to improve their complexions, when in fact the roughness and soreness of their skin is a symptom of mild scurvy, which could be cleared up by spending a fraction of the beauty budget on blackcurrants or oranges.

People who have lived in hot countries and move to a colder latitude need to make a positive effort to increase the amount of vitamin D in their diet. Where the sunshine is strong and custom allows people to expose their bodies to it, most of the necessary vitamin D is created in the skin itself by sunlight, and the amount in the diet is often very low. If such people move to a country like Britain, where the amount of sunshine is less and the human body has to be similarly shrouded, it is more necessary to get the vitamin from food—margarine, butter, milk, eggs, fish, and so on. Many immigrant families in Britain suffer from some degree of rickets because of this vitamin deficiency. This is especially so among Indian and Pakistani girls, who are required to keep themselves almost entirely covered from top to toe.

Those who eat a lot of carbohydrate—sugar, starch, etc.—or drink a good deal of alcohol, are obviously laying up other troubles for themselves, but in particular need more vitamin B_1 than the average, to help them metabolize the energy food. Folic acid is also more essential to the heavy drinker than the abstainer. Many of the symptoms put down to alcohol poisoning are really signals of vitamin B group deficiency in the alcoholic.

The problems of vegans, who do not eat any animal products, and therefore tend to be short of vitamin B_{12}, have already been considered on page 55 in describing the problems experienced by Bernard Shaw when following such a diet.

'*Natural Foods*'   Strangest of all the magical beliefs about diet that are canvassed among the diet reformers, is the idea that everything 'natural' must have been designed by providence to be entirely suitable for man. The writer of the article on dolomite, mentioned earlier, was obviously convinced that the proportions of calcium and magnesium in this particular limestone must be exactly right for the delicate balance of the human metabolism, because it was 'natural'. He ignored, apparently, the fact that the composition of dolomite was originally intended for making up shells for generations of prehistoric molluscs, whose fossil remains now form the great limestone cliffs, and that these creatures might have had their own requirements for the ideal proportions of calcium and magnesium in their protective shields.

However, 'if it's natural it must be safe' seems to be a motto that survives any amount of contrary evidence. As has been said above, even vitamins can sometimes be poisonous if they are taken to excess, yet I have seen this very phrase used as a headline for an article assuring health-food users that it is impossible to have too much of good things like vitamin pills. As for plant foods, even a cursory consideration will show that the number of natural products which are acutely harmful to man is very great indeed.

The *Solanaceae* family alone, for instance, should be convincing proof that natural is by no means safe. They appear to have been designed by a rather homicidal providence to be both attractive and noxious in their effects. Deadly, woody, and black nightshades are some of the more notorious members of the family, with their appetizing bright berries filled with atropine and other poisons, but henbane, thorn-apple (Jimson weed), tobacco with its deadly extract nicotine, and several other killers are also related. Even the edible members of the family such as the potato are by no means entirely safe: the green sprouts of seed potatoes contain the poison solanine which has been known to kill unwary diners. In World War I a company of hungry German soldiers found some seed potatoes and boiled them whole to get a quick meal of soup: they all died of solanine poisoning. The tomato and the aubergine are also *Solanaceae*, and it is at least feasible that the old traditions that these fruits were poisonous, or harmful if eaten raw, may have had some foundation of truth—in many cases the harmful characteristics of the wild or semi-cultivated varieties of plant have been bred out by generations of artificial selection. The case of lettuce, apparently one of the mildest of plants, is considered in the next chapter (pp 125–6).

Many other plant toxins exist, of which the most dramatic are some of the toadstool poisons in plants such as *Amanita phalloides*, the Death Cap, or *Boletus satanas*, the Devil's Toadstool, both of which look very much like varieties of harmless edible fungi. Many vetches and peas contain *lathyrus* poisons that can cause malformation of the bones if they account for a large proportion of the diet, and mustard oil, an essential cooking oil in many parts of Bengal and Bihar, sometimes contains oil from the seeds of a weed *Argemone mexicana*, so poisonous that even traces of it can cause epidemics of dropsy among the population. Doctors spent years looking for unknown bacterial or virus diseases as a cause of the illness before it was traced to a 'natural' additive in the diet.

The ackee fruit, common in Jamaica, is attractive and quite appetizing, but it must not be eaten in any large quantities, otherwise it causes a 'vomiting sickness' very like bacterial food poisoning or dysentery. Cycad nuts can cause liver damage and even cancer.

Many foods, while not strictly poisonous in themselves, are undesirable components of diet because they destroy or interfere with essential vitamins and minerals from other foods. Large quantities of raw cabbage, a popular food among food reformers, interfere with the uptake of iodine by the thyroid gland and can thus cause goitre even when iodine is present in the diet. Some fish, such as carp, pike, perch and bream, contain an 'antivitamin' that destroys the activity of thiamin, vitamin B_1, and thus induces a deficiency disease like beriberi. Clovers sometimes cause dangerous or fatal bleeding in cattle by interfering with the action of vitamin K, the 'blood-clotting' vitamin. In the next chapter some even stranger actions of natural foods are recounted.

The logic of the 'natural equals safe' school of thought is tenuous, and the actual principle behind it is suspiciously like the anthropocentric belief that everything on this earth or in the skies was designed purely for man's benefit or entertainment:

Be fruitful, and multiply, and replenish the earth, and subdue it; and have dominion over the fish of the sea, and over the fowl of the air, and over every living thing that moveth upon the earth. And God said, Behold, I have given you every herb bearing seed, which is upon the face of all the earth, and every tree, in the which is the fruit of a tree bearing seed; to you it shall be for meat. (Genesis 1, 28–9)

Unfortunately it seems that Nature has not read the text properly, and man's dominion over large numbers of fish, fowl, animals and plants is rather shaky. Each species develops with the primary aim of ensuring its own continuance, and many plants and fish, in particular, have secured their own safety by becoming extremely poisonous to possible predators, including man.

The whole idea that plants or animals were created to serve man is, in fact, sublimely arrogant, and Nature has devised some bizarre ways to punish that arrogance, as may be seen in the next chapter.

9 Food for Thought

Apart from a few dedicated mechanists, most people will accept that the human mind has a considerable degree of control over the workings of the body. Evidence comes from all sides that the controls of the body machine can be overridden by the brain: healing by a variety of faiths, whether the faith is religious conviction or just the belief that the doctor's pills must do something, the very real control exercised by yoga adepts over their heartbeat, digestion, and other so-called involuntary functions, the superstitious fear that often literally kills victims of a witch-doctor's curse, or those who break a taboo. There are even such everyday examples of mind-control as the will that gets an extra effort out of the tired muscles of athletes or travellers if the challenge is important enough. The study of such mind-control, bio-feedback, is a very fashionable exercise.

But although we call it bio-*feedback*, implying a two-way traffic, we seem unwilling to admit that the body can equally control the mind. Try telling someone that his righteous anger is really only a product of indigestion, or that his political beliefs are a symptom of thyroid deficiency, and you will receive a very dusty answer. We retain an intellectualist conviction that our thoughts and beliefs are purely rational, not swayed by the unknown tides of the body and its organs, and the idea that the food we eat could have a direct effect on our thinking is extremely distasteful.

However, as with mind-control, evidence for body-control is all round us. How often have we met someone who is irritable to the point of violence before dinner, but mellows almost visibly as he forks in the food? Jerome K. Jerome, in *Three Men in a Boat*, devotes one of his inimitable parentheses to this aspect of human nature:

> It is very strange, this domination of our intellect by our digestive organs. We cannot work, we cannot think, unless our stomach wills so. It dictates to us our emotions, our passions. After eggs and bacon, it says, 'Work!' After beefsteak and porter, it says, 'Sleep!' After a cup of tea . . . it says to the brain, 'Now, rise, and show your strength. Be eloquent, and deep, and tender; see, with a clear eye, into Nature and into life; spread your white wings of quivering thought, and soar, a god-like spirit, over the whirling world beneath you, up through long lanes of flaming stars to the gates of eternity!'
>
> After hot muffins, it says, 'Be dull and soulless, like a beast of the field . . .'

Jerome's light-hearted comments would have seemed entirely reasonable, indeed self-evident, to the medieval dietitians who adopted the doctrine of humours as the basis for their recommendations. Whatever its faults as a foundation for a medical science, the doctrine took it for granted that the human organism must be treated as a 'whole man', in which mind and body were equally affected by the prevailing humour and any alterations in it induced by diet. It also got away from the notion, so widespread in modern nutritional writing, that one kind of diet is equally suitable for people of all ages and dispositions. The doctrine not only divided individuals into the four basic types of sanguine, phlegmatic, choleric, or melancholic, but allowed for changes in the ruling type brought about by ageing or circumstances—thus children were considered to be, in general, phlegmatic until puberty, becoming then more sanguine or choleric, according to physical and psychological type. When old age slowed down the vital processes, the person became phlegmatic again.

Diet was chosen to suit the dominant humour, and its effects were expected to be seen equally in the body and the mind. For example, lettuce was classified as cold and moist, the qualities of the phlegmatic humour, and would therefore produce a cooling and slowing down not only of the body and its functions, but also of the temperament. Eating lettuce was therefore recommended not only for feverish conditions, which were obviously hot and dry and demanded to be treated with cold and moist food, and for opening the bowels, another physical attribute of the 'phlegmatic' foods, but for regulating the choleric (hot and dry) high spirits of lusty young men. Sir Thomas Elyot, in *The Castel of Helth* (1539), says, 'Yonge men, exedyng the age of xiiii. yeres, shal eate meates more grosse of substance, colder and moyster: also salades of cold herbes . . .', and Culpeper, in his *Herbal*, makes the real point plainer by commenting, on lettuce, that 'it abates bodily lust, represses venereous dreams . . .'.

Similarly, food classified as cold and dry was considered suitable fare for those of a sanguine (hot and moist) temperament, but would produce melancholy if eaten in excess, especially by people of a naturally melancholic or phlegmatic disposition. Thomas Muffet warned that venison was only suitable for the sanguine—'Galen numbreth it amongst hard, melancholique, and gross Meats'—and James Hart in *Klinike* claimed that the same was true of many game birds, particularly the waders—'Snite or snipe engender melancholy, as do heron, storke, crane, bustard, and bittour [bittern]'. A little earlier Robert Burton, in *The Anatomy of Melancholy*, had listed a whole catalogue of foods to be avoided if melancholy was to be kept at bay:

All venison is melancholy, and begets bad blood . . . Hare, a black meat, melancholy, and hard of digestion . . . Milk, and all that comes of milk, as butter and cheese, curds, etc., increase melancholy (whey only excepted, which is most wholesome) . . . Amongst fowl, peacocks and pigeons, all fenny fowl are forbidden, as ducks, geese, swans, herons, cranes, coots, didappers, waterhens, with all those teals, currs, sheldrakes, and peckled fowls, that come hither in winter out of Scandia, Muscovy, Greenland, Friesland, which half the year are covered all over with snow and frozen up. Though these be fair in feathers, pleasant in taste, and have a good outside, like hypocrites, while in plumes, and soft, their flesh is hard, black, unwholesome, dangerous, melancholy meat.

And so on. Burton's diatribe rumbles on, like a juggernaut, for two more pages of condemnation of fish, 'cold' vegetables such as cucumbers and gourds, roots, onions and garlic, pears, apples . . .

While, as usual with Scholastic sciences, the doctrine of humours represented an enormous superstructure of fanciful deduction based on a very shifty and shallow foundation of fact, there are many points of truth and accurate observation in among the fantasy that must have served as convincing evidence that the doctrine was working in practice, especially in the absence of any alternative medical theory worthy of the name.

Modern writers are inclined to lose patience with the extravagances of the doctrine, especially when set out by compulsive word-spinners like Burton, and to dismiss the whole literature on humours as so much fantastic nonsense. This does less than justice to the writers and doctors who supported and used the theory. Elyot, Burton, Muffet, Hart, Culpeper and so on were not fools, and their writings often show a sharp practical sense of observation. However, like modern doctors, they had their successes and their failures, and like modern doctors, they were inclined to ascribe the successes to sound theory and medical skill, and their failures to bad luck. Often it turns out that their theories had more than a spice of truth in them, even when they sound strange to modern ears.

For example, the use of lettuce as a kind of anaphrodisiac or tranquillizer may seem odd to those of us who think of lettuce as a pleasant but rather dull foundation for salads. However, the medieval and Tudor lettuce would not have been as highly developed as the modern garden lettuce (*Lactuca sativa*), and more like the coarser and larger wild lettuce, *Lactuca virosa*. The milky juice of this plant actually contains substantial amounts of materials such as lacturin, lactucopicrin, and allied compounds that behave as a mild narcotic. The dried resin, called Lactucarium, was used until quite recently as a gentle sleeping draught, safer and less habit-forming than opium products or barbiturates, and it is still apparently found from time to time as a completely unauthorized addition to real opium. The wild lettuce is sometimes called the 'opium lettuce', and the dried Lactucarium looks and smells so much like opium resin that it can fool an expert.

This behaviour of wild lettuce accounts for the numerous references in modern herbals and books on natural medicine to the use of lettuce as a tranquillizer or cure for insomnia. Some of these are obviously copied uncritically from the older books. In particular I have seen in at least four modern herbals the peculiar, and quite incorrect, statement that the milky juice of lettuce is laudanum (tincture of opium). There is, as so often in these older remedies, a basis of fact if only it can be un-covered. Perhaps Beatrix Potter was thinking of the old tradition when she imparted to the readers of *The Tale of Peter Rabbit* the useful information that 'lettuces are very soporific': at least this must have ensured the continuance of the belief among generations of children who might never have read a herbal.

Incidentally, those who enjoy garden lettuce need not be too concerned lest they fall into a coma over their plate of salad: while it is true that *Lactuca sativa* contains a small amount of the narcotic material, you would have to eat several pounds of lettuce per meal before it had any pharmacological effect: equally it does not seem necessary to set up a special Lettuce Branch of the Drug Squad to prevent furtive orgies of lettuce eating. However, when garden lettuces run to seed, the unpleasant bitter taste of the fleshy stem is probably due to lacturin and its allied compounds. The taste is so nasty, however, that no one would be likely to eat very much of the stem.

As we have seen in the previous chapter, natural products are not naturally safe to eat, whatever the food reformers say, and many of them contain drugs that affect the mind or personality. Most people know about the narcotic and poisonous properties of the nightshade family, henbane, water-hemlock (cow-bane), thorn-apple (Jimson weed), and so on, although there are still too many cases of accidental or self-inflicted poisoning every year from these and similar plants. Children are attracted by the large juicy berries of deadly and woody nightshade, especially as these flourish after most of the other soft fruit has disappeared from the hedgerows, but the atropine in the fruit causes hallucinations, emotional disturbances, and a general sense of loss of touch with reality. Large doses can cause coma, death, or permanent eye damage. Atropine is still used in ophthalmic work as eye-drops to widen the pupil, and up to Victorian times fashionable ladies used to put it in their eyes to make them look dark and luminous (as *extract of belladonna*) until it was realized that the repeated use of the drug imposed such a strain on the eyeball that their sight was ruined.

Henbane and thorn-apple, which both contain hyoscyamine and scopolamine (hyoscine, the 'truth-drug'), have occasionally been eaten by accident. Henbane smells so unpleasant that it cannot often have been taken, but thorn-apple or Jimson weed looks and smells quite edible. There is an amusing account of the first contact of British soldiers with Jimson weed in Virginia in 1676. After eating it with other strange green vegetables some of them behaved as if 'pursued by devils', while others clowned about. All of them remembered nothing of this when they recovered.

Mostly these plants are eaten or smoked by people in search of a new thrill, and they usually get more of an experience than they expected, because the hallucinations from these drugs can be very terrifying—monsters, demons, and the whole repertoire of nightmares. The paranoia and feelings of persecution may persist for days—if the experimenter recovers at all.

However, apart from these known poisons, there are quite a few common foods that have psychotropic effects, even though they are normally considered harmless. For example, *lathyrism* is a name for a series of diseases caused by various vetches or pulses. One such plant is the chickling vetch (*Lathyrus sativa*), known in India as *khesari dhal*. This is not much grown in Europe, but is an important 'insurance' crop in India and the Middle East. Farmers sow a mixture of the vetch and wheat:

if the rains are abundant the wheat soon overgrows the vetch, which dies down and furnishes a useful source of nitrogen for the growing wheat. If the season is too dry for wheat, the hardier vetch grows to full size and can be harvested as an emergency food crop.

Mixed with other kinds of *dhal* (lentils, pigeon peas, and so on), khesari is harmless, and indeed a useful source of protein. However, if times are hard and khesari is the only available food, people soon develop nervous troubles, a feeling of lassitude and depression, and often symptoms like acute alcoholic intoxication. This obviously plays its part in hindering better farming methods, and in fact can ruin community life. The 'loco weed' that drives horses and cattle mad in the drier states of the USA is a similar plant, and there is a plant called *miscara* in the Middle East (the flax darnel, *Lolium temulatum*) which occasionally gets into wheat fields in Ethiopia and Aden, and, if ground up with the wheat and made into bread or porridge, can cause acute intoxication, even in small quantities. This may explain the extreme suspicion of vetches or 'tares' in Biblical times—'But while men slept, his enemy came and sowed tares among the wheat.' (Matthew, 13, 25)

Hydrogen cyanide (prussic acid) and cyanides occur quite widely in foods, and, even if not concentrated enough to kill, can cause intoxication and the father and mother of all hangovers. The lima bean (a kind of butter bean or sugar bean, *Phaseolus lunatus*) sometimes accumulates enough cyanide for a quarter of a pound to be the lethal dose, and almonds, peach and plum stones, and apple pips all contain cyanide, enough to cause serious effects from time to time. In the south of France, the old and heroic method of making the liqueur *prunelle* was to fill a wooden cask with plums, nail the lid on, and leave the fruit to ferment for six months. The result, distilled from the remains, was possibly the most potent liquor since the time of Lucrezia Borgia. One glass was almost a passport to a lost weekend, mainly because of the potent effects of the various organic cyanides formed from the plum stones during the long fermentation. There is still a liqueur called *prunelle*, but it is a pale modern imitation of the traditional product.

Some narcotic poisons can get into our food second-hand, so to speak. There is a great deal of concern today about the build-up of pesticides and other artificial poisons in the bodies of animals that eat chemically-treated grass, and so on, but the same process has been going on naturally for centuries. Quail, for example, can apparently feed on poison hemlock without the slightest ill-effect to themselves, but in doing so they stuff their flesh full of coniine—the alkaloid in hemlock that finally silenced Socrates—so that people who eat the birds develop double-vision, difficulty in walking, and all the other symptoms of drunkenness.

Bees have been known to collect nectar from poisonous flowers and turn it into honey that causes visions, giddiness, and even convulsions. The ancient Greeks and Romans, who depended a great deal on honey as their only source of sugar, imported it from all round the Mediterranean, and soon got to know that some supplies were suspect. Xenophon, in the *Anabasis*, warns his readers against honey from Trebizond, where it is often made from the nectar of a plant he calls *Aegolethron*—probably *Rhododendron ponticum*, as many of the rhododendron and azalea family can give rise to poisonous honey without apparently harming the bees or their grubs. Pliny, in his *Natural History*, has a section about the intoxicating honey imported from Persia and parts of Morocco.

Natural stimulants can have even worse effects than the narcotics, if they provoke people to violent and anti-social acts. For example, the toadstools Fly Agaric (*Amanita muscaria*) and False Blusher (*Amanita pantherina*) both contain myco-atropine, a drug that produces acute intoxication even if quite small quantities of the fungi are eaten, and, according to the experts, 'violent and hilarious' moods. In Lapland and Eastern Siberia, where alcohol is hard to come by, the inhabitants make Fly Agaric into a drink guaranteed to turn any solemn assembly into a riotous party. This beverage was obviously of great use to while away the long Lapp winter, and Catherine the Great is reputed to have arranged for supplies of the product to be sent from Siberia to the imperial palace to liven up that already farouche institution. She became extremely fond of the stimulating effects herself, and often became wildly hilarious—a rather terrifying development in such a despotic empress, one would imagine.

Similar fungi containing mycoatropine form the 'Sacred Mushrooms' eaten in various parts of the world, in primitive societies and misguided 'civilized' ones, to induce violent religious fervour. The hallucinations caused by the drug are accepted as ecstatic religious illuminations, just as many other mystical experiences can be traced to psychotropic drugs. Unfortunately most of the fungi that contain mycoatropine, which affects the mind, also contain muscarine, a simple and effective poison. Many people have ended up in hospital with muscarin poisoning because they have eaten the showy red and white Fly Agaric to get 'high'.

The False Blusher causes even more accidents, because it looks like an ordinary brownish mushroom, and many innocent collectors have picked and eaten the dangerous fungus in mistake for the tasty and harmless Blusher (*Amanita rubescens*). As the False Blusher contains more of both drugs than Fly Agaric, fatalities are common.

Among the most familiar food products with stimulant effects are the various plants that produce beverages—tea, coffee, cocoa, maté, cola, guarana, and so on. Almost every part of the world has some stimulating plant of the kind, and there has been a trade in them from ancient times. Most of the plants contain caffeine (called theine in some older books—it took some time for the chemists to find out that the drugs in tea and in coffee were in fact the same material), mixed with the milder stimulants theophylline and theobromine. Cocoa, as befits its tamer reputation, contains only theobromine.

The lively effects of these drinks were discovered and exploited very early. The Chinese traditionally date the discovery of tea to the Emperor Shen-nung in 2737 BC, but even if this is entirely mythical, there is no doubt that tea was in use in parts of China some centuries before the birth of Christ. Another charming myth of its origin, which explains the value placed on it as a stimulant and reviver, is that the monk Bodhidharma vowed to spend nine sleepless years contemplating the virtues of Buddha, but could only stay awake by chewing the leaves of a nearby shrub, the tea plant.

Coffee was in use in Turkey by at least AD 1000, and again it was prized for its stimulating effects, especially in a society debarred from alcohol as a social lubricant. As Robert Burton explains in *The Anatomy of Melancholy*:

> The Turks have a drink called coffa (for they use no wine), so named of a berry as black as soot . . . they spend much time in these coffa-houses, which are somewhat like our alehouses or taverns, and there they sit chatting and drinking to drive away the time, and to be merry together, because they find by experience that kind of drink, so used, helpeth digestion and procureth alacrity.

Sir Thomas Herbert, writing in 1626, had more to say about the restorative action of coffee:

> There is nothing that the Persians do love more than the 'cohs' or 'copha', called by the Turks 'capha'. This Drink seems to derive from the Styx, as it is so black, thick and bitter. It is said that it is healthy when drunk hot . . . It destroys melancholy, dries the tears, softens anger and produces joyful feelings.

Once the drinks were introduced into Europe, it was not long before people became aware of the 'lift' that they could bring. Coffee houses sprang up all over London during the ten years following the establishment of the first one in St Michael's Alley in 1652, and all of them soon served not only coffee, but chocolate and tea: 'That excellent and by all Physitians approved China Drink called by the Chineans *Tcha*, by other nations *Tay, alias Tee*, is sold at the Sultaness Head, a cophee-house in Sweetings Rents, by the Royal Exchange, London' an advertisement of 1658 runs. In 1660 Pepys wrote in his diary, 'I did send for a cup of tee (a China drink) of which I never had drunk before'.

During the eighteenth century tea, in particular, became the main stimulant for the working people of Britain. They soon found out that a cup of tea could warm and cheer them even when the rest of their diet was near starvation level, and the tea helped to wash down stodgy meals of bread and cheese. Sir Frederick Eden, in *The State of the Poor* (1797) was surprised by the fact that families with barely forty pounds a year to spend on food would lay out two pounds on tea, and Arthur Young (*The Farmer's Tour Through the East of England*, 1771) noted that when the inmates of a House of Industry were allowed twopence out of every shilling they earned to buy extra food, they invariably bought tea and sugar.

Robert Tressell, with a closer personal acquaintance of starvation conditions, describes the value of tea to the poor in *The Ragged Trousered Philanthropists* (about 1906):

> They still had credit at the baker's, but they did not take much bread: when one has had scarcely anything else but bread to eat for nearly a month one finds it difficult to eat at all. That same day . . . they had a loaf of beautiful fresh bread, but none of them could eat it, although they were hungry: it seemed to stick in their throats, and they could not swallow it even with the help of a drink of tea. But they drank the tea, which was the one thing that enabled them to go on living.

This sinful indulgence in stimulants did not go uncriticized, of course: Eden called tea 'this deleterious produce of China', and Jonas Hanway (*An Essay on Tea*, 1757) asked vehemently, 'When will this evil stop? Your very *Chambermaids* have lost their bloom, I suppose by *sipping tea*.' Many modern writers on diet condemn the taking of drugs in the form of tea, coffee, and cola drinks. Dr Henry G. Bieler, in *Food is Your Best Medicine* (1968), leaves no doubt that coffee is an addictive poison, and draws a horrifying picture of the coffee-junkie trying to cut down:

> Instead of feeling better instantly, he finds himself wracked (sic) with a constant and violent headache. He is surprised when told he is suffering withdrawal symptoms, milder to be sure, but still symptoms like those a narcotics addict suffers.
> The headache following coffee withdrawal persists for the

length of time it takes the coffee poisons to be eliminated . . .
After the body is made toxic by a high concentration of coffee
poisons over a long period of time, coffee ceases to stimulate,
no matter how much is drunk, and a period of depression
follows . . .

Dr Bieler, not a man for half-measures, then goes on to
prophesy arthritis, neuritis and cancer for the unregenerate
coffee drinker. The fact that none of his dire warnings on the
dangers of coffee are true (except perhaps for someone drinking
twenty or thirty strong cups per day) is irrelevant: what comes
over is his passionate *moral* objection to the stimulating properties of caffeine.

Dr Robert C. Atkins, of the famous Diet Revolution (see
page 147) makes similar comments about coffee and tea
addiction, rather complicated in his case by the fact that he
does not seem to know that caffeine is the main stimulant in
tea.

Despite the protests of such writers, the use of caffeine as a
stimulant is increasing. Apart from tea and coffee, and the
popular South American beverages maté and guarana, caffeine
is added to many soft drinks—the *cola* from which they take
their name is hardly ever used now, but equivalent amounts of
caffeine from tea-dust, etc. are added. Caffeine is added to many
common drugs such as aspirin to overcome the depressing
effects of the drug and the illness (the universal APC tablets—
aspirin, phenacetin and caffeine—use up tremendous quantities
of the drug).

For those who genuinely find that caffeine keeps them awake
at night, or, like the Mormons, prefer to avoid all stimulants,
decaffeinated coffee is widely available. Many health-food
writers recommend this as somehow more healthy than the
drug-saturated natural product—an odd attitude for people
who usually spend a great deal of space criticizing modern
'mass-produced' foods because they have had their 'vital
principles' removed during processing. One would have thought
that caffeine is coffee's only 'vital principle'—without it the
drink is just a rather burnt-tasting brown fluid.

While caffeine and its related compounds are relatively mild stimulants, some common foods can accumulate far more potent drugs. Nutmeg, for instance, contains myristicin, similar to LSD in its effects on the brain, and as little as a fifth of an ounce of the powdered spice can cause hallucinations and a feeling of exhilaration, followed by deep depression the next day. Bananas, especially when very ripe, contain enough adrenalin, serotonin, and other mental stimulants to cause serious disturbances. Small amounts of these substances are essential for the working of the brain and nervous system, but an overdose, as can occur in communities where bananas have to be the main source of food, causes irritability, violent and irrational reactions to the most innocent actions or comments, and a state bordering on mania.

However, without doubt, the stimulant drug that has produced the most dramatic and tragic results is ergot, a fungus ('rust') that attacks rye and some other cereals. This mould grows on ears of rye, gradually taking over the grains and replacing the starch by a dark, hard mycelium. If this is ground up with the rye grains and passes into flour, anyone eating the rye product will develop ergotism. One form of this starts with a burning feeling in the extremities (St Anthony's Fire) and leads to gangrene and loss of fingers, toes, or even whole limbs. The more usual reaction is a kind of dancing madness, with hallucinations and convulsions.

This is hardly surprising, as the ergot drugs are closely related to LSD, and the same symptoms are reported—many people suffering from the drugs were killed or injured in falls from rooftops, as they were convinced they could fly, others suffered terrifying visions of demons or monsters pursuing them. A very widespread outbreak of ergotism occurred in Central Europe at the same time that the Black Death (bubonic plague) was devastating the area, and the madness then took the form of bands of half-crazy people moving from village to village flagellating themselves and describing the visions that they could see. Often the flagellants died from their self-inflicted injuries, but in the general atmosphere of terror during the Black Death, when it must have seemed that the Angel of Death was walking the streets, most people accepted these deaths as a kind of human sacrifice that might even conceivably keep the plague away from their village or town. The dreadful mortality had stripped away the superficial layer of Christianity in Europe, and most people had reverted to magic in an attempt to drive away the disease, often killing or banishing scapegoats to 'send the Death away', so the wild drug-induced ceremonies of the flagellants must have seemed at least as useful as the prayers and fasting of the clergy.

In Britain the amount of ergotism was far less than in the rest of Europe, because so little rye was grown or eaten regularly. In times of shortage imported rye sometimes brought the disease (the last big outbreak of ergotism in Britain, 200 cases in Manchester in 1925, was due to imported rye), and very occasionally other cereals were attacked. In Wattisham in Suffolk in 1762 the family of John Downing, 'a poor labouring man', was attacked by ergotism, and the local surgeon, Dr Wollaston, was interested enough in this case of *Raphania*, as ergotism was then called, to note down details of their diet, and in particular the fact that they had eaten no rye bread. The disease was finally traced to a batch of sub-standard wheat sold off cheaply by a local farmer.

It is clear that there are many components of food and drink that can affect our minds profoundly, and that these turn up in some of the most innocent foodstuffs. What about *shortages* of essential nourishment? It emerges that these also have a direct effect on our thoughts and feelings, and perhaps a more insidious one. It is possible to find out about poisonous or psychotropic drugs in foods, and avoid those foods if we want to stay clear of the drugs, but when a mental state is caused by a deficiency of something in our diet, it is far harder to find out what that missing something is.

Starvation, or the shortage of all types of nourishment, invariably causes severe mental changes. The first signs are personality recession: the hungry person becomes querulous, easily irritated by trifles, and restless. Simple tasks become too much trouble, and efforts by outsiders to help in any way are usually rewarded with a snarl. It is as if the hungry body had reduced the mind to that of a food-hunting animal. One of the first lessons learned by members of the emergency services who are called in to deal with famine and other cases of mass-starvation is that they can never expect to be thanked for anything they do, however noble or kind. The starved person is not capable of such a reaction.

The accounts of the potato famine in Ireland during the 'hungry 'Forties' make tragic reading, but one of the most disheartening features of them is the evidence of petty quarrelling, abortive fights over nothing at all, and the general disintegration of generous and cheerful personalities into food-grubbing grumblers. Accounts of life in Japanese prisoner-of-war camps in World War II show the same personality breakdown under starvation conditions.

The second set of changes is even stranger. Hallucinations begin, first, naturally enough, of food, but soon the visions become more general. Here one can only suppose that the dying body is trying to surround itself with at least the semblance of a new life. These hallucinations, in religious communities throughout the world, have been taken as actual glimpses of some mystical reality, and fasting, carried out originally merely as an exercise in subduing the body, became a passport to mystical experience.

'Pleasure and guilt are synonymous terms in the language of the monks, and they had discovered, by experience, that rigid fasts and abstemious diets are the most effectual preservatives against the impure desires of the flesh', comments Gibbon in Chapter 37 of *The Decline and Fall of the Roman Empire*, and goes on to describe the consequences of this fasting,

> Their visions, before they attained this extreme and acknow-ledged term of frenzy, have afforded ample materials of supernatural history. It was their firm persuasion that the air which they breathed was peopled with invisible enemies; with innumerable daemons, who watched every occasion, and assumed every form, to terrify, and above all to tempt, their unguarded virtue. The imagination, and even the senses, were deceived by the illusions of distempered fanaticism;

and the hermit, whose midnight prayer was oppressed by involuntary slumber, might easily confound the phantoms of horror or delight which had occupied his sleeping and his waking dreams.

A century and a half before, Burton had also launched a characteristic diatribe against the use of fasting to procure religious visions:

> Never any strange illusions of devils amongst hermits, anachorites, never any visions, phantasms, apparitions, enthusiasms, prophets, any revelations, but immoderate fasting, bad diet, sickness, melancholy, solitariness, or some such things were their precedent causes ... "tis a miraculous thing to relate' (as Cardan writes) 'what strange accidents proceed from fasting; dreams, superstition, contempt of torments, desire of death, prophecies, paradoxes, madness; fasting naturally prepares men to these things.' Monks, anachorites, and the like, after much emptiness, become melancholy, vertiginous, they think they hear strange noises, confer with hobgoblins, devils ...

Fasting is indeed a very useful exercise for any religion that requires absolute faith from its followers. The subjugation of the body satisfies the sense of guilt that drives most of the acolytes into the stranger sects, and, as we have seen so often in dietetic systems, food is a universally recognized symbol of bodily indulgence. The fact that even a moderate degree of starvation brings its religious reward in the form of visions, illuminations, mystical experiences and glimpses of absolute truth is a bonus that few religious leaders can afford to ignore. Perhaps the most bizarre of the fasting cults was that of Heydon, one of the leaders of the Rosicrucian movement in Britain in the seventeenth century. Heydon believed that eating was mankind's original sin (not just eating the fruit of the Tree of Knowledge, but any food). He insisted that for the faithful the air would provide all the nourishment needed, and that the hungry could be satisfied merely by placing a plate of cooked meat on the stomach and inhaling the aroma.

Apart from gross starvation, shortages of some apparently minor ingredients of food can lead to very odd mental states and even madness. For example, it has been recorded in Europe for centuries that communities using maize as their main source of food tended to be afflicted by a disease which started with reddening and roughening of the skin. It was accordingly called *pellagra* (Italian *pelle agra*=harsh skin). Soon, after this first symptom, more serious changes occurred— the sufferers developed diarrhoea and pains in the stomach, and became thin and ill. Worst of all, they began to suffer from hallucinations, personality changes, and all the signs of incipient madness. Early doctors characterized pellagra by 'the 3 Ds—dermatitis, diarrhoea, and dementia'.

Many investigators noticed the strong resemblance between pellagra and ergotism, and supposed that there was some similar but undetected poison in the maize: 'A disease in Italy has been ascribed to the long-continued use of maize as a food, but it is not certain whether it is not rather due to a fungus attacking the maize, than to the use of pure maize.' (Alexander Blyth, *Diet in Relation to Health and Work*, 1884)

While pellagra was being investigated as an interesting curiosity in Europe, it was becoming a way of life in the southern United States. Around the turn of the century, the South was a one-crop region, depending almost entirely on cotton for its economic survival, and the standard of living and eating was incredibly low for white and black alike. Many poor sharecroppers needed all their land for cotton, and could not grow much food for themselves, and the millhands in the towns fared even worse. The general diet consisted of corn meal and grits, soda biscuits, corn syrup, and fat salt pork, and even when they had enough bulk of food, the Southerners developed sore skin and mouths, became thin and listless, and suffered from depression, hallucinations, irritability, and other mental disorders.

This clinical description of the typical poor Southerner, any time between about 1900 and 1940, comes alive in the novels of William Faulkner—the brooding sullenness suddenly shattered by outbursts of irrational anger, persecution mania, the feeling of people living in a cruel and demented world of their own. Hundreds of victims of pellagra were in fact herded into lunatic asylums, and there must have been thousands more whose behaviour was unstable or disturbed, while not quite mad enough for the asylum. Novels like Faulkner's *The Sound and the Fury* must be the nearest approach that most of us will have to the disordered world of the chronic pellagra sufferer.

Doctors knew very well that diet was at the bottom of all the misery they saw around them, and that the disease could be kept at bay by a balanced food supply. As Drs Wheeler and Sebrell wrote in 1932:

> In looking for cases of pellagra, the home surrounded by evidence of a good garden, or a cow or two, a few pigs and some poultry, may as well be passed up, for the chances are less than one in a thousand that pellagra will be found. On the other hand, the home surrounded only by last year's cotton patch will always bear watching.

The Red Cross distributed dried yeast, already noted as a cure for the disease, or could sometimes lend a rural family a cow until the general health and earning power had improved, but it was not until 1937 that it was finally proved that pellagra was due to a shortage in the diet of the very simple compound nicotinamide. Although known to chemists as a breakdown product of nicotine since about 1867, it had not been recognized as an essential food component. Nicotinamide shares none of the properties of nicotine, but organic chemists tend to run out of names for compounds, and therefore lump together materials having nothing in common except their chemical 'skeleton'. However, to avoid confusion with nicotine, the Americans call the vitamin *niacin*. Goldberger, who discovered its action, called it the *P-P factor* (pellagra-preventive), and in older books it is sometimes referred to as vitamin B_5 or B_3, but these names are obsolete and are usually only found in 'health-food' literature.

The discovery that such a simple material could have such profound effects not only on the body but on the mind set off a great wave of nutritional research. One mystery was soon solved: doctors had known for years that poor Mexicans who also lived mainly on maize might suffer from many other diseases, but very rarely from pellagra. It emerged that there was in fact some nicotinamide in maize, but in a form that could not easily be absorbed. The Mexican women had a custom taken from traditional Indian food preparation, of soaking the corncobs in lime water before they made their *tortillas*. This apparently released the vitamin. It is an ironic thought, that the adoption of one simple 'primitive' custom might have saved the tens of thousands of ruined lives in the Southern states.

Soon it was discovered that less of the vitamin was needed if there was plenty of protein in the diet, and particularly protein containing the essential amino-acid *tryptophan*. This knowledge might not have helped much in the worst periods of pellagra, because the people were too poor to buy much protein, and tryptophan is one of the rarest of the amino-acids. However, it did explain why foods like milk and eggs, low in actual nicotinamide but rich in tryptophan, could keep pellagra away. Nutritionists now total up the nicotinamide and tryptophan and talk about the *nicotinamide* (or *niacin*) *equivalent* of foods.

In recent years gross pellagra has almost disappeared. It is very simple to treat, either with food rich in the vitamin, like yeast, or with synthetic nicotinamide, that can be made so cheaply that the required daily dose of the vitamin costs only pennies. Now doctors are looking at the fringe effects, and in particular seeing whether some types of mental illness or depression may be due to a slight shortage of nicotinamide or tryptophan. The latter is particularly interesting in its effects on the brain, as it is converted in the body to tryptamine and serotonin, two materials which have extraordinary effects on the brain—too little causes sluggishness, depression and stupidity, too much causes over-excitement and irritability. Good results with some types of schizophrenia have been obtained simply by feeding the patients with a diet rich in nicotinamide and tryptophan, and many people suffering from depression, or what Robert Burton would have called 'melancholy', are now being given tryptophan, either by adding the pure material to other food, or just by selecting a suitable diet, instead of the far more dangerous tranquillizers manufactured by the pharmaceutical companies.

Sir Arthur Conan Doyle, in *A Medical Document*, puts into the mouth of one of his characters the true horror of the tight-rope which all of us walk between sanity and madness:

> Is it not a shocking thing . . . to think that you may have a fine, noble fellow with every divine instinct, and that some little vascular change, the dropping, we will say, of a minute spicule of bone from the inner table of his skull on to the surface of his brain may have the effect of changing him to a filthy and pitiable creature with every low and debasing tendency. What a satire an asylum is on the majesty of man.

One feels he would have made the same point about the effects of the microscopic traces of vitamins or poisons in our food. A pin's head too much ergotoxin in our rye bread, and we leave reality for a lunatic world peopled by Hieronymus Bosch monsters, where we can fly: a pinch of nicotinamide missing from our food, and we become morose, suspicious, surrounded by a host of imaginary enemies. We are not merely the slaves of our stomachs—we are brainwashed by them.

10 Rituals
for the Global Village

One of the major results of the modern explosion in communications is that we are all constantly fed with snippets of information about the traditions, customs, and cultures of other parts of the world. In Africa or south-east Asia, people know about the latest Western gadgets or fashions almost as soon as the New Yorker or Londoner, and in return we in the West are continually reminded of exotic customs, medicines, foods, or systems of thought that contrast in a colourful way with our normal background.

Obviously we rarely get enough information about these things to understand the deeper significance of them, but there are dozens of exegetists only too ready to produce a kind of *Readers' Digest* condensation—two or three thousand years of a culture distilled down to a handful of platitudes. We are given the froth on the surface of an alien system of thought, but rarely permitted to explore the depths underneath.

For example, while only about one person in a million in the West really knows very much about the traditions or methods of Chinese medicine, popular texts on acupuncture appear on every bookstall, and this one small facet of the Chinese system is inflated to a cult. Similarly the Hare Krishna movement provides a highly-coloured picture book version of Vaishnava Hinduism, but with only a very superficial reference to the complex and profound body of Hindu theology. Earnest students and bored housewives tie themselves up in yoga postures learned from TV lessons and expect all the wisdom of the East to enter into them automatically.

Exotic diets become fashionable in the same way. The Krishna followers go to immense trouble to produce food acceptable to the god and his consort Scrīmratī Rādhāraṇī, and unfortunately the gods are so chauvinistic in their tastes that only traditional Indian food will do, so one finds pleasant but solemn young men and women scouring the shops of Denver or Watford for asafoetida and mango powder, *urad dhal* and gram flour, to make a sort of Americanized version of ordinary Indian cooking. In the same spirit they may be found turning perfectly good butter into ghee (clarified butter-fat)—not, as in India in the past, because that is the only way to preserve the butter without a refrigerator, but because ghee is part of the ritual of preparing food for Krishna. Curiously enough, as refrigerators become more common in India, the need to make ghee from butter is becoming less acute, and more people are using the butter unclarified.

But such logical points are not the central nexus of the worship of Krishna. One might wonder why, if the god is a universal power, he could not be content with offerings of well-made indigenous food—why, for example, the English Hare Krishna follower should not offer a Yorkshire pudding made with loving care—but this is not the appeal. The real charm of the Krishna diet is essentially that the ingredients are hard to obtain and the food is unlike indigenous American or English food, just as the robes, bare feet, and shaven heads of the followers stand out from the normal dress of their contemporaries. The diet is, in fact, a ritual, and as such satisfies a deep psychological need for ritual and ceremony in the Krishna followers.

Similar considerations apply to the macrobiotic diet, introduced by Nyoiti Sakurazawa (George Ohsawa as he calls himself in his American books) from Japan into the USA, and thence to the whole of the Western world. Macrobiotics depends on a diet mainly of grains—brown rice, wholewheat, barley, rye, oats, millet, buckwheat, and so on—with beans of all kinds and a few vegetables. In a similar way to the classifications adapted in Europe when the doctrine of humours controlled medicine and diet, foods in macrobiotics are classified into yang, or masculine, foods, and yin, or feminine, foods, and with a sexist bias worthy of all the best traditions of Japan yang foods are in general considered superior.

As with the doctrine of humours, there are vast ramifications of theoretical thought built up on the simple foundations of yin and yang. One table of yin and yang properties runs as follows:

Yang	*Yin*
Light	Dark
Hot	Cold
Dry	Moist
Hard	Soft
Masculine	Feminine
Active, creative	Passive, receptive
Animal	Vegetable
Contracted, small	Expansive, large
Heavy	Light
Red, orange, yellow	Green, blue, purple
Salt, bitter	Sweet, sour, peppery
Alkaline	Acid
Sodium	Potassium

Obviously such a list of antinomies is a marvellous toy to play with, and writers on macrobiotics can fill pages of their books with lists of yang foods and yin foods, choosing any combination of the qualities that can be made to fit in with the actual nature of the diet. But, when you get down to details, it turns out to mean very little. What, for example, is the status of lemons, which are yellow (yang) but sour (yin)? Is carragheen moss yin because it is green, or yang because it is one of the very few vegetables to contain more sodium than potassium? Things get worse when writers try to give quantitative lists. I have one before me that classifies fruit from the most yang (apples) to the most yin (huckleberries), and I have yet to discover any rational basis for the order, even assuming the list of qualities above. For example, blackcurrants are near the top of the list, and therefore yang, but they are sour and contain a very large excess of potassium over sodium (the ratio is about 1:135), which ought to make them yin. On the other hand, melons are near the end of the list, which implies that they are yin—but melons have a ratio of potassium to sodium of only 1:23, and are mostly red or yellow, both yang characteristics.

One excuse for such gross nonsenses is to say that everything has a balance of yin and yang—an idea reminiscent of the old apologists for the doctrine of humours, who used to explain the anomalies in their system by mixtures of the various humours. On the rare occasions, however, when by accident a food happens to possess all the qualities necessary to make it fully yin or yang, it is surprising how quickly the idea of balance gets forgotten.

Of course, the ritual value of the macrobiotic diet does not depend on its very shaky philosophical basis, but, as with the Krishna movement, on the appeal of its exotic ingredients. The mainstay of the diet is traditional Japanese cooking slightly modified for western use, with grains and various types of bean as the bulk of the meal. Bread made with prepared yeast is not common in Japan, so the macrobiotic dieter has to return to the 'sourdough' method that was common in Europe and America a century ago, leaving the dough to collect 'wild' yeasts from the air until it rises. This is a perfectly reasonable method, except that other organisms can float into the dough and produce mouldy bread at least, and food poisoning if you are unlucky. However, whatever is Japanese is right, for the macrobiotic. Similarly European flavourings and sauces are considered as poisons, because they might contain artificial flavouring ingredients, but the Japanese sauces *miso* and *tamari*, made by fermenting soya beans, are not only permitted, but insisted upon. As both of these materials, though tasty, are full of monosodium glutamate, it seems odd to find them in a diet dedicated to the elimination of 'chemical' ingredients.

However, most people would say, 'Why not let them get on with it?'—the fact that a diet is nonsensical or illogical is no reason to condemn it if people like to follow it. This seems reasonable enough: if anyone likes to adopt a Japanese diet and pretend that it is doing them good, this is no worse than joining those comic groups of people who dress up in ten-gallon hats and chaparajos and pretend to be cowboys, or the Hare Krishna followers who dress up in Indian robes, eat Indian food, and pretend to be Hindus. Unfortunately, the macrobiotic diet is not only useless, but positively harmful. The rules of the diet, which preclude meat and discourage fruit and most vegetables, lead to a serious shortage of vitamin C. Many dedicated followers of the system have in fact developed the early signs of scurvy. If you follow some of the more extreme gurus of macrobiotics you may fare worse than this. The American Academy of Paediatrics published a paper in 1977 showing that some of the more rigid macrobiotic systems practised in the USA can lead not only to scurvy but low protein and calcium levels in the blood, anaemia, emaciation, and eventual death, virtually from starvation.

Writers on the diet tend to make matters worse by pretending that, if dieters become ill, this is due to 'accumulated poisons' working their way out of the system, and not to the fact that the diet itself is harmful. There is a Catch-22 approach in the literature—if you feel good on the diet, that is entirely due to the magic of macrobiotics but if you feel ill, that is the result of your previous bad eating habits. Consequently many people put up with bouts of nausea, indigestion and weakness, confident that everything will get better when they have been on the diet long enough, until at last they make themselves really ill and need medical treatment.

An example of this doublethink is contained in a little book by Craig Sams, *About Macrobiotics*: 'After the first few days [dieters] may become groggy or ill as poisons accumulated from years of unbalanced eating are released into the blood stream to be carried away.'

An even more heroic approach is taken by the book *Get Well Naturally*, by Linda Clark: 'Acute illness should, therefore, be regarded as a remedial and beneficient outlet, rather than something to be feared or suppressed.' The same approach is used in many dietetic systems, as for example in the apology for the dreadful effects of the Grape Diet already quoted on page 79. In general, if a diet makes you feel ill, the best thing to do is to stop immediately. This principle has saved countless people from doing themselves real harm with some of the crazier systems suggested in the world of fringe medicine. This applies particularly to diets for losing weight—another semi-religious ritual in most western countries.

For example, Dr R. C. Atkins's *Diet Revolution*, which has been spread all over the global village by modern mass communication, is a system that satisfies the most desperate need for ritual and sacrifice. Simplified to its actual effect on your eating habits. Dr Atkins's theory is that you can lose weight drastically without feeling hungry if you cut out carbohydrates of all kinds (starches, sugars, and so on), but fill up with unlimited amounts of fatty foods—cream, mayonnaise, bacon, eggs, fried meat, rich cheese, etc. The idea is, as Dr Atkins says himself, to achieve a deliberate imbalance in the diet, so that the body can only maintain its energy levels by breaking down fat, and in doing so uses up the fat in your bulges as well as that in your diet.

This idea is not new—it has been in use for years under the name of the *ketogenic* diet, because in the unbalanced state the body produces substances called ketones from the excess of fat (acetone, a common solvent for lacquers, is typical of the ketone family). These ketones appear in the urine when the state of *ketosis* starts, and one of the more bizarre rituals of Dr Atkins's diet is testing your urine with a special test paper called Ketostix, hoping to see the paper turn purple. Unfortunately the ketones also appear on your breath, giving it a smell of rotten apples, and they tend to produce giddiness and nausea (just as acetone will, if you breathe it in unwisely).

These last two sets of symptoms had the expected effect in most cases of making people give up the diet before they had done much harm to themselves. A typical personal report was given by reporter Valerie Wade in *The Sunday Times*:

> After seven faithful days, I was 5 pounds lighter, without the slightest twinge of hunger, had experienced extreme nausea and practically vomited in the street, and was worried about bad breath . . . I have since met very few people who kept

up the diet for more than two self-possessed weeks. (21 October 1973)

The American Medical Association was worried about more than bad breath and nausea. They declared Dr Atkins's diet 'unscientific and potentially dangerous to health'. Dr Frederick J. Stare of Harvard wrote that '. . . any diet which tends to be high in saturated fats and cholesterol tends to elevate the chance that the individual will get heart disease. Any book that recommends unlimited amounts of meat, butter and eggs, as this one does, is in my opinion dangerous'.

The ketosis that occurs is similar in many ways to the state into which diabetics get if their supply of insulin is cut off or irregular. They too have the ketones in their urine and breath, and smell of rotten fruit. They also suffer from giddiness and loss of control, to such an extent that there have been many cases of quite sober diabetics being arrested for drunkenness. As the ketogenic diet, the system was in fact used in the twenties as a possible palliative for young people with epilepsy—someone had noticed that children who were both diabetic and epileptic very rarely had fits when they were in the ketosis state, and some doctors recommended artificially-induced ketosis as a treatment. If the choice before you is ketosis on the one hand or epileptic fits on the other, there is some justification for trying the diet (although it does not seem to work very well): for normal people it seems fraught with unnecessary dangers.

However, despite all the disadvantages, the diet was very popular for a time, and still crops up from time to time in the form of food systems that allow you to eat fat but not starch or sugar. The rituals were ideal for middle-class people with too much time on their hands—searching the supermarkets for the most nauseatingly rich foods, with Dr Atkins's charts clutched in your sticky little hand, peeing on a test paper in the hopes of seeing it turn purple, watching your acquaintances admire your sylph-like figure (though from the safe distance required by your bad breath). As with so many other diets, Dr Atkins somehow contrived to discount the unpleasant symptoms by suggesting that these were the results of your previous bad eating habits (the old 'poisons working their way out of the system' routine).

The ketogenic diet was unreliable, but had a sound physiological basis—it really reflected the reactions of the body to excess fat. A more common (and much safer) way of inventing a new diet system is to give sound, middle-of-the -road advice that can do nobody any harm, but trick it out with some new, crazy 'scientific' or mystical principle that will ensure that your diet gets full publicity from all the newspapers and women's magazines. A typical example is the so-called 'magnetic diet' advanced by Michel Gauquelin, Director of the splendidly-named Institute for the Study of Relationships Between Cosmic and Psycho-Physiological Rhythm in Strasbourg. Dr Gauquelin's diet amounts to no more than increasing the mineral and fibre content of your food, an idea which is hardly original, but is at least safe enough. To make this a little more complicated, he has tables of foodstuffs from which you must get the various minerals, but, strange to say, these are mostly correct—while some foods that contain a particular mineral are not mentioned, at least the ones that are listed really do provide a source.

So far, so good, except that such a commonsense system would not rate a paragraph in any national journal. Gauquelin's stroke of originality is to claim that all of the minerals he recommends are magnetic, and that therefore every human cell that contains them will respond to the great magnetic tides of the earth, magnetic storms, sunspots, and 'the whole rhythm of the universe'. By eating more minerals you make yourself more magnetic, and so by some unspecified process more lively and attractive to the opposite sex.

Whether or not there is any truth in the science fantasy about magnetic rhythms in the universe, their influence on most of the minerals mentioned by Gauquelin would be negligible. Iron and cobalt are quite strongly magnetic, but some of the others, such as iodine, are practically non-magnetic, or at least far less magnetic than even the water which composes the greater part of the body.

The 'magnetic diet' is thus no more than a piece of entertaining nonsense, but at least a few days, or even a few weeks, devoted to it will do you no real harm, and might even slightly improve your health and figure if your normal diet is of the 'chips with everything' type. New systems of this kind spring up all the time—astrological diets, with foods related to the signs of the zodiac, diets with complicated points systems, like bridge scorecards, vitamin boosters, high-fibre diets, and so on —but as long as they are not too expensive to keep up and give you a basic mixture of fresh foods, without excess of any one dietary component, they do very little harm, and can be regarded as just another trendy game to play—if you have that sort of time to spare.

More important are the occasional entries into the 'health food' arena of the large food manufacturers, characterized by a massive public relations campaign and a tendency to play down any disadvantages of the chosen product for the slimmer. Such a campaign was the 'Slimming *with* Bread' diet of a year or two back. Bread has a bad name among slimmers, who represent a growing proportion of the population, partly because of its high calorie value, and also because of the numerous attacks on white bread by food reformers. In any case, bread tends to have a decreased sale as societies become more affluent and have greater access to a variety of alternative foods.

All these factors made the flour manufacturers realize that bread would have to be rehabilitated. An expensive advertising campaign was launched to remind people that even white bread contains vitamin B_1, calcium and iron, all valuable nutrients. This was backed up by little booklets directed at slimmers, mothers of young families, and various other groups. Their justification for bread as a slimming food was a little tortuous— of the two main sources of calories, fats or starch (the message ran), most people found it harder to give up starch. So, it followed, it was better to eat bread and cut down on fat, and be fairly satisfied, than to reduce the bread, eat fat, and still feel empty.

However, there were a few insignificant facts that somehow got left out of the advertisements and even the booklets . . .

One of these missing facts, a strange omission in such a detailed survey of the dietetic value of bread, was its calorie count. One slice of a medium-sliced white loaf rates about 92 calories, so the average UK consumption of six slices per day would contribute 550 calories—quite a proportion of the 2,500 calories or so used up by the average person in Britain. If you were trying to slim by maintaining a calorie-controlled diet of about 1,250 calories a day, six slices of bread would use up almost half your allowance—even if you ate them dry. The slightest smear of butter or margarine to help them down would add another 30 calories per slice, or 180 during the day, making 730 in all. Not perhaps the best foundation for a low-calorie diet. Admittedly, bread contains valuable minerals and vitamins, but if you want to slim you would do better to get these from vegetables, which do not contain so much starch.

When a newspaper commented on this curious feature of the campaign, the Flour Advisory Bureau reportedly replied, 'There isn't anything sinister about this. It's just the way it came. We don't actually spell out the number of calories.' And, sinister or not, the public were left with the impression that bread was not fattening, whatever the small print might say.

A similar campaign was run to boost the sales of Guinness stout, another product of which slimmers have a healthy suspicion. As the Guinness brewers were trying hard to promote their product to women, they obviously felt that the slimming angle would be the best approach, and came out with the seven-day Guinness diet. To be fair to the advertisers (and one feels quite sure that they worked hard to encourage such fairness to them), the whole campaign was more tongue-in-cheek than the bread promotion, and the 'seven-day diet' did not go in for boring old figures. But again the crucial information, the calorific value of the recommended product, was entirely missing from the newspaper advertisements or the detailed leaflets.

Possibly this omission had just a little to do with the fact that a pint of Guinness contributes 220 calories to your intake, as many as if you had eaten 10oz of boiled potatoes, which no slimmers in their right mind would contemplate for a moment.

In the actual diet leaflet it was made clear that you must restrict yourself to one half-pint of Guinness at lunchtime, and another in the evening, but anyone not reading the small print, and simply assuming that Guinness was a slimming drink, could easily find themselves putting on weight with alarming speed—six pints a day would use up the whole allowance of a calorie-controlled diet before you even had a bite of food.

This sort of incursion into the world of slimming and health diets merely brings Big Business into more disrepute than it already enjoys, and the magazines that deal with wholefoods, nature cures, and similar food reform systems are not slow to point out the fact. In the same way these magazines are constantly criticizing the large food groups for forcing convenience foods, additives, white sugar products, and similar things on the public. Sometimes one sees the suggestion that the orthodox medical profession fail to recognize whatever the latest wonder diet may be, because of sinister pressure from these same big food companies.

What is conveniently forgotten in these diatribes is that the health food business itself is large and powerful—about $800 million turnover per annum in America, £50 million in Britain —and the profit margins on health foods are often very much higher than those on 'conventional' foods in the local supermarket. For example, wholefood cornflakes sell at prices at least 50 per cent higher than those of Big-Business Kellogg's cornflakes, while in fact the mass-produced product is rather more nutritive than the 'natural' one, because Kellogg's add vitamins to their flakes. Similarly, bulk muesli sold in a health-food shop cost 42p per pound when an almost identical product made by a large milling group cost 22p per pound. The profits on 'tissue-salts' as mineral supplements have already been hinted at (page 113). In a typical health store vitamin tablets worth, at the very most, 10p retail for over 100p.

Such uncomfortable facts do not weigh very heavily with the users of these stores, mainly because buying health foods has very little to do with health or food. A diet is not just a system for eating but one of a group of social, ethical, or even political beliefs and aspirations. Like your books, furniture, hobbies and clothes, your diet is a declaration of a set of attitudes to the world, whether consciously or unconsciously.

The quest for 'wholefoods', for example, uncontaminated by pesticides, artificial fertilizers, additives, or modern packaging, has very little to do with the nutritional value of the food, but a lot to do with a conscious rejection of the methods and values of the Big Businesses that provide the pesticides, fertilizers, additives and packaging material. This is a diet that projects a militant 'socially conscious' image, and tends to go with political activism and a fair degree of innocence of the world. The sad thing is that if you have a perfectly justifiable suspicion of 'Big Business food' you tend to find yourself automatically lumped together with these political innocents in all their other attitudes. 'I don't go into vegetarian shops,' I can recall one intelligent vegetarian telling me, 'You meet such awful people there.'

Diet and attitudes to the world go together just as surely in the case of the conventional eater. The stolid conservative man (it is usually a man) who rejects any variation in his chosen diet of beef, potatoes and pudding, may be expressing more than a dietary resistance to change. It may be a deep distrust of all the ways in which the world is changing round him. The Sunday joint may be, for him, a symbol of all the solid virtues that are being eroded by modern life. The sudden appearance of a soya-bean stew in its place would be an insult not only to his digestion, but to Queen and Country.

I have restricted the subject of this book to attitudes to diet, rather than diet itself, but it must be clear by now that diets are symbols of beliefs that existed long before the food reforms themselves were conceived. Seneca and Ovid started off with a conscious rejection of the gross sensuality of Roman life around them, and gradually rationalized this into the cult of the simple life and vegetarianism. Muffet and the other philosophers of the Doctrine of Humours treated diet as if it were just one aspect of the grand design which they longed to find in the whole scheme of existence, with man as God's highest creation and everything in the universe planned for his use and comfort.

The early vegetarians of the nineteenth century, such as Shelley, tried to reverse this attitude, and push man out of his self-appointed place at the centre of the cosmos. Their rejection of meat was a recognition that animals were not created solely for man's use.

So on through the ages, attitudes to diet have reflected the popular ethos of the time, or a reaction to it. The modern emphasis among dieters for 'back to the land' simplicity and a rejection of all the advantages of food technology is just one symptom of a widespread feeling of disillusion with science and technology in general—while at the other extreme the modern health-food store with its pills, potions, 'magic' foods and expensive diet supplements is part of the great market machine for extracting money from the consumer for a continuous flow of new products.

The most striking characteristic of modern diet, in the west, is the degree of choice that exists, partly because of the amount and variety of food available for most of the population, and partly because of the rapid dissemination of every new diet-system by the mass media. The choice of diets, of rituals and sacrifices, has never been greater or more bewildering, and it is not surprising that people find themselves confused by the barrage of dietary information and misinformation which confronts them. I hope that this book has cast a little light on some of the more opaque mysteries of the diet scene, and that it may enable some people to choose a regime that suits them, physically and temperamentally, without falling for the charlatanism that is so often associated with discussions on food.

There is no ideal diet—every person's needs, tastes, and metabolism are different. All that one can try to do is to follow the path of moderation, what the Buddha called the Middle Path, and avoid the two extremes: 'Sensuality is low, vulgar, worldly, ignoble, and conducive to harm; self-mortification is painful, ignoble, and conducive to harm. The Middle Path avoids these extremes and gives vision, gives knowledge, and leads to peace, insight, enlightenment, and Nirvana.'

Appendix

A Few Facts and Figures

There are, scattered through this book, numerous items of nutritional information that were intended to illuminate particular points—usually to show whether older theories were right or wrong by the standards of modern nutritional research. Some readers would no doubt like to have these stray facts rounded up into a tidy arrangement, and this also gives me the opportunity to quote authorities and sources for the opinions I have expressed, without overloading the main text with references and figures.

However, I should like to make clear two points about this small glossary of nutritional terms:

a It is not intended to do more than skim the surface of a very large subject. Readers who want to explore further will find a select bibliography on pages 167–72. Experts will, I hope, forgive a certain amount of simplification of points of detail.

b I do not advocate any particular diet or food supplement, except the usefulness of a well-mixed diet with plenty of fresh food. Where I say, for example, that a certain vitamin or trace element is known to be essential for the health of the eyes, skin, and so on, this does not imply that food containing such materials will cure disorders. Any abnormality, however slight, should be referred to a qualified medical practitioner. It is worth recalling, also, that there are over 200 *known* inborn abnormalities of the digestive system which make certain foods unsuitable for some people, and only an expert can diagnose these.

Amino-acids are the 'building blocks' from which proteins are made up. There are about twenty-four different types commonly found. The digestive system breaks down protein foods into the individual amino-acids, which can circulate in the bloodstream, and these are then put together in different combinations to form protein where it is needed, for the muscles, skin, hair, and so on. They also play an important part in the nucleus of the cell and in hormones such as insulin.

Some of the twenty-four amino-acids can be converted into others in the human body, but others have to be obtained from the food we eat. These are called *essential amino-acids*—eight different ones are needed for adults and two extra for infants. These are listed under their own names.

Arginine is one of the essential amino-acids for children: it is widely distributed, and ample amounts can be obtained from milk and eggs. A shortage slows down growth.

Ascorbic acid is another name for vitamin C, because it cures scurvy.

Biotin is a vitamin (once called vitamin H). A deficiency causes loss of hair, dermatitis, and general weakness. However, most normal diets provide plenty of the vitamin, and it can also be produced in the digestive system. Raw white of egg interferes with this vitamin, and in fact the only authentic case of 'natural' deficiency was in a food fanatic who ate 9 dozen raw eggs per week. The recommended daily intake is 0.15–0.3mg for an adult. Liver and kidneys are particularly good sources.

Calciferol is another name for vitamin D, because it is essential for incorporating *calcium* into bones.

Calcium, phosphates, and vitamin D are needed to make calcium phosphate, which forms the hard skeleton of bones. A lack of any of the three materials can make the bones soft (rickets) or brittle (osteoporosis). Very young and very old people tend to suffer more from these diseases because of inadequate diet. Hard water can supply almost half the necessary daily intake of calcium—in soft water districts it is necessary to find other sources. The recommended intake for adults is 400–500mg per day: a pint of milk will give more than this.

Carbohydrates are the main sources of energy for the body: sugar and starch are used in this way by man and several other animals, but ruminants and rodents can also digest the carbohydrate cellulose from grass, tree-bark, and so on. In man cellulose acts as non-digested fibre.

All carbohydrates, when digested, are broken down into sugars that can be used immediately for energy, or stored in the body as glycogen or fat. The recommended daily intake of 3,000 calories (12.5 MJ) for a normal adult could be provided by 760g (just over 1½lb) of sugar, or 850g (nearly 2lb) of pure starch such as cornflour, but these would furnish absolutely no other nutrients. In fact, many adults and children actually eat more than this amount of sugar or starch every day, and thus make themselves overweight and lose their appetite for more nourishing food.

Carotene is one form of vitamin A, so called because it was first discovered in carrots.

Cholesterol is a waxy solid that occurs mainly in fatty foods— eggs, brains, and fat meat contain considerable amounts, butter and full-cream cheeses are other sources. While it is a natural component of the fats in the bloodstream, some authorities think that excess cholesterol causes blockages in the blood vessels and hence ischaemic heart disease (IHD). A diet rich in polyunsaturated fatty acids (qv) seems to lower cholesterol levels and therefore reduces the risk of IHD: the American Heart Association recommend that polyunsaturated fatty acids should form 11–14 per cent of the total energy intake, and that cholesterol from foods should be reduced to 300mg per day (or about 3 egg yolks per week) where there is a serious risk of IHD. However, some equally-qualified doctors think that the risks are exaggerated.

Choline is a vitamin of the B group, not normally in short supply in any adequate diet, as it can be formed in the body from proteins.

Chromium is a normally poisonous metal, but its compounds are needed in very small quantities to ensure reliable metabolism of sugars. Old people on a generally inadequate diet often suffer from chromium deficiency. It is found in particular in wholegrain foods and seafoods.

Cobalamin is another name for vitamin B_{12}, because it contains *cobalt*.

Cobalt is another trace *element*, whose compounds are needed for control of the metabolism. It forms part of the vitamin B_{12} molecule, but as this has to be obtained ready-made from food, it is probable that other forms of cobalt are useless for human diet (although sheep seem to be able to use the simple cobalt compounds applied to their grass).

Copper, like chromium, is poisonous in large quantities, but is needed in traces to ensure blood formation. About 2mg per day seems to be the required level: a normal well-balanced Western-type diet provides up to 5mg, but in case of deficiency, liver or dried fruit are good sources.

Essential amino-acids are dealt with under their individual names.

Essential fatty acids or **polyunsaturated fatty acids** are linoleic acid, linolenic acid, and arachidonic acid, found combined in most vegetable and fish oils, but not so much in animal fats. A certain minimum quantity of essential fatty acids (sometimes called *vitamin F*) is needed for proper skin growth, but their importance has increased with the theory that they may also be connected with the amount of cholesterol in the bloodstream (see *Cholesterol*). It is important to note that frying in vegetable oils reduces the essential fatty acids by up to 30 per cent.

Fats are the main other energy food beside carbohydrates. Solid fats like suet, and liquid fats like peanut oil, vary only in the *fatty acids* they contain. Some (vegetable oils and fish oils) contain more *essential fatty acids* than others, but apart from this you can calculate that 325g (about ⅔lb) of any fat will give you *all* of the 3,000 calories (12.5 MJ) needed per day. As many foods, such as confectionery items, contain fat and sugar together, it is obviously easy to exceed the recommended energy intake and convert the surplus to fat in the body.

Fibre is mainly cellulose, which human beings cannot digest. It serves a useful purpose in giving the intestines something solid to move, and for this reason some people eat bran and other cellulose food wastes. With a normal diet this is un-necessary: the bran naturally present in wholemeal bread is quite sufficient for normal purposes, and if wholemeal bread is not liked, the cellulose in raw fruits and green vegetables will usually suffice.

Fluorine is essential for the production of healthy tooth enamel, and a shortage causes rapid decay. In many districts the water supply contains enough soluble fluorides (about 1 part per million) for the teeth: where this is lacking the best solution is to add sodium fluoride to the water to make it up to the required level. This is opposed on moral grounds by some groups, but the scientific evidence they advance is often based on misunderstandings (for example, great play is made of the fact that sodium fluoride in concentrated form is poisonous—the same could be said of copper and many other materials essential to the body in small quantities). Fluorides are difficult to get from food sources alone; only seafoods usually contain enough to make up for shortages in the water supply.

Folic acid is a vitamin of the B group, necessary for a number of body functions, including blood formation. Fortunately it is widely distributed in food. About 0.4mg per day is necessary for adults. In cases of deficiency the richest sources are liver, oysters, and green vegetables such as asparagus, spinach, and turnip tops. Overcooking is bad for this vitamin, and over 50 per cent can be destroyed by lengthy boiling.

Iodine is necessary for the hormones of the thyroid gland, and hence for properly balanced growth. In most places there is enough iodine, in the form of soluble iodides, in the water supply, but in some mountainous districts—for example, Switzerland and Derbyshire in England—the natural amount is so small that the thyroid gland swells to produce *goitre* ('Derbyshire neck'). Some foods, such as beans and cabbage, can actually interfere with the thyroid function, and cause goitre if eaten to excess, even when there is iodine in the diet. The best way to remedy a shortage is to use iodized table salt, or to eat seafoods or seaweed (kelp) preparations.

Iron is necessary to form the red corpuscles in the blood, and a shortage can cause anaemia (although this is not the only cause: blood formation also requires adequate vitamin B_{12}, vitamin C, folic acid, traces of copper, and possibly cobalt). The World Health Organization recommends about 12mg per day for most adults, and 18mg per day for women of child-bearing age. As the *average* UK diet only contains about 12mg of iron per day, many people are getting less than they need. Cereals supply most of the iron (in many countries, including the UK, iron salts are added to flour to ensure that the level is kept up), meat, eggs, and potatoes are other good sources. Black treacle (molasses) contains about 9mg of iron per 100g (41mg per lb), mostly dissolved out from the processing machinery when it is manufactured. Iron, like most other minerals, is not affected by cooking.

Isoleucine is one of the essential amino-acids. The average adult should have about 1.4g per day: this could be obtained from 100g (just under ¼lb) of cheese, about the same amount of lean beef, or 112g (¼lb) of lentils.

Leucine is another of the essential amino-acids. The average adult should have about 2.2g per day: this could be obtained from 100g (just under ¼lb) of cheese, slightly more lean beef, or 130g (4½oz) of lentils.

Lipoic acid is a fat-soluble vitamin that is essential for all metabolic processes. Fortunately it is widely distributed in all types of food, and deficiencies have never been recorded under normal circumstances.

Lysine is an essential amino-acid that is needed for growth. The average adult should have about 1.6g per day: this could be obtained from 82g (about 3oz) of cheese, 73g (about 2½oz) of lean beef, or 110g (about ¼lb) of lentils. Lysine tends to be lost during drying and high-temperature cooking, so correspondingly more food is necessary to give the recommended amount.

Magnesium is a mineral essential for metabolism. About 250mg per day is necessary for the average adult, and as magnesium is present in chlorophyll any green vegetables will give ample supplies—so will pulses such as lentils and beans. Alcoholics sometimes suffer from magnesium deficiency due to a generally poor diet.

Manganese is another mineral, also necessary for metabolism, but only in trace amounts, about 5mg per day, which can easily be obtained from almost any diet.

Menaquinone is another name for vitamin K (qv).

Methionine is an essential amino-acid, necessary for the correct working of the liver, and for many other processes, such as the replacement of skin and hair cells. The average adult should have about 2.2g a day: this could be obtained from 370g (13oz) of cheese, 340g (12oz) of lean beef, or 1,400g (about 3lb) of lentils. It is clear that methionine is rarer than most of the other essential amino-acids, and it does in fact take a good deal of thought to get enough of it from a purely vegetable diet.

Monosodium glutamate is a compound of one of the non-essential amino-acids, glutamic acid, and is released from meat proteins during cooking. It is one of the substances that accounts for the 'savoury' taste of cooked meat, which used to be called *osmazome* (see page 69). Monosodium glutamate can also be obtained by fermenting vegetable materials, such as sugar-beet residues and soya beans, and it occurs in large amounts in soy sauce, miso, and tamari, which can therefore be used to give vegetable meals a 'meaty' taste. It is used in large amounts to flavour soups and tinned meats, etc, and while this may make such foods rather monotonously the same in taste, there is no evidence that it does any harm.

Nicotinamide (niacin) is a vitamin of the B group. A deficiency of it causes pellagra (see pages 138–41). The vitamin is widely distributed in meat and vegetables, but not so much in dairy products. The UN Food and Agriculture Organization recommends about 16mg per day for an adult: this could be obtained from 100g (just under ¼lb) of liver, 400g (14oz) of mushrooms, etc. Diets that contain a lot of millet or maize may be deficient in nicotinamide. It is one of the most stable vitamins, and is hardly affected by cooking, canning, freezing, or drying.

Pantothenic acid is another vitamin of the B complex (once called B_3, but not now) and is essential for the proper working of the nervous system. Fortunately, as its name suggests, it is present in practically all types of food, so deficiency is extremely rare. The recommended intake (US National Research Council) is about 10mg per day: 100g (about ¼lb) of liver or 200g (7oz) of broad beans would supply this. Cooking and canning can destroy up to 50 per cent of the pantothenic acid in foods, freezing does less damage.

Phenylalanine is an essential amino-acid needed for production of hormones and other body functions, including the formation of hair colour. The average adult should have about 2.2g per day: this could be obtained from 172g (6oz) of cheese, 200g (7oz) of lean beef, or 220g (½lb) of lentils.

Phytic acid is a component of bran and other fibrous material, such as the skins of broad and other beans. It can combine with calcium and iron in some foods and make them unavailable to the body, which is one of the reasons for enriching flour with calcium and iron salts. However, there are mechanisms by which phytic acid can be broken down (the yeast in bread, for example, does this to some extent).

Polyunsaturated fatty acids (see Essential Fatty Acids).

Potassium is essential for all the energy systems in the body. As it is regularly excreted, there is a constant need for replacement at a rate of about 3g per day. Many old people actually get far less than this. Milk and cheese are good sources of the mineral.

Proteins are needed to repair and build up all the tissues of the body. About 40–50g should be eaten daily, including the essential amino-acids (qv). Where the diet contains too little protein, but a lot of carbohydrate, children get a wasting disease called *kwashiorkor*.

Pyridoxine is another name for vitamin B_6 (qv).

Riboflavin (sometimes called vitamin B_2) is needed for many cell systems. The UK Department of Health recommends 1.7mg per day for average adults, and it is certain that a good many people get less than this. One pint of milk *and* 170g (6oz) of cheese would furnish the right amount, but it is important to note that riboflavin, though fairly stable to cooking, is destroyed by light, so milk should not be left on the doorstep or window-sill.

Thiamin is another name for vitamin B_1 (qv).

Threonine is an essential amino-acid: the average adult should have about 1g per day, which could be obtained from 85g (3oz) of cheese, about the same weight of lean beef, or 115g (4oz) of lentils.

Tocopherol is another name for vitamin E.

Tryptophan is an essential amino-acid which is important because it can make up for shortages in nicotinamide. The average adult should have about 0.5g a day: this could be obtained from 140g (5oz) of cheese, about the same amount of lean beef, or 260g (9oz) of lentils.

Valine is the last of the essential amino-acids. The average adult needs 1.6g per day, which could be obtained from 90g (just over 3oz) of cheese, 112g (4oz) of lean beef, or 120g (just over 4oz) of lentils.

Vitamin A is a fat-soluble material which is essential for the well-being of the eyes. The first symptom of deficiency is night-blindness, which is followed by xerophthalmia, an unpleasant drying of the eyes. The daily intake for adults should be about $750\mu g$ (2,500 International Units), which could be obtained from 72g ($2\frac{1}{2}$oz) of butter, 83g (3oz) of margarine, or about 135g ($4\frac{1}{2}$oz) of carrots. The body can store a certain amount of the vitamin from one day to another, but an overdose can be poisonous (see page 116). The vitamin is fairly stable to cooking, except roasting or drying, and to canning or freezing.

Vitamin B$_1$ or **thiamin** is necessary for many parts of the metabolic system, and the deficiency disease appears as the nervous complaint *beriberi*. The UN Food and Agriculture Organization recommends a daily intake of about 1.2mg, which could be obtained from 600g (just over $1\frac{1}{4}$lb) of wholemeal bread, or similar cereal products. Eggs, liver, and fish roe are also good sources. The vitamin is widely distributed, but tends to be destroyed by cooking and canning, and, as it is soluble in water, can be thrown away down the sink if vegetables are boiled in a lot of water.

Vitamin B$_2$ is riboflavin (qv).

Vitamin B₆ or pyridoxine is important in many reactions that occur in the body. Fortunately it is so widely distributed that deficiency is almost unknown. The recommended daily intake is about 2mg, which could be obtained from 500g (about 18oz) of wholemeal bread or 200g (about 7oz) of brazil nuts. About 35 per cent of the vitamin, on average, is destroyed during cooking or canning.

Vitamin B₁₂ or cobalamin is essential for blood formation, and a shortage causes pernicious anaemia. The vitamin is widely distributed in meat and dairy products, but very rare in vegetables and fruits, so people on a purely vegan diet have problems (see pages 55–7). The recommended daily intake is about 1μg, which could be obtained from as little as 2g (0.07oz) of liver.

Vitamin C or ascorbic acid is essential for the health of the blood vessels and skin, and for a number of other body reactions. Lack of it causes *scurvy*, shown first by bleeding gums, then bruises and bleeding in the skin: wounds take a long time to heal, and old ones may suddenly open up again. The US National Research Council recommend a daily intake of 60mg per day, while the UK Department of Health recommend only 10mg per day. Taking the midway figure of 35mg, this could be obtained from 17g (just over ½oz) of raw blackcurrants, or 200g (7oz) of boiled new potatoes. In fact, potatoes are the main source of the vitamin in the UK diet.

The vitamin is easily destroyed by overcooking, oxidation (for instance, by chopping up vegetables and then leaving them exposed to the air for a long time before cooking), during canning, and to some extent during freezing, so it is only too easy to get less than enough vitamin C if you live on 'convenience' foods or depend on an inefficient canteen or restaurant.

Professor Linus Pauling, winner of two Nobel prizes, has claimed for some years that, apart from the avoidance of scurvy, taking very large doses of vitamin C (several grams per day) can prevent colds and other illnesses. This has not been convincingly proved or disproved. It is not necessary to use large quantities of fruit or vegetables for such dosage, as the vitamin can be made by fermentation methods on a large scale.

Vitamin D or **calciferol** is needed for bone formation. It is fat-soluble, like vitamin A, and can be stored in the body, but again like vitamin A it can be poisonous if taken in large quantities. The vitamin is formed in the skin when exposed to sunlight, so you do not need as much intake from food if you get enough sun: conversely, if you live in a bad climate or swaddle yourself in concealing clothes (as, for example, women living in purdah) you need extra supplies of the vitamin in food. The recommended intake for an adult in the UK is about 2.5μg (100 International Units) per day: this could be obtained from 33g (just over an ounce) of margarine, or 250g (about 9oz) of butter.

The vitamin is not much affected by cooking, such as frying.

Vitamin E is the name given to a group of materials called *tocopherols*. It seems to be essential for the maintenance of membranes in man: in some other animals it is essential for fertility. The vitamin is widely distributed, particularly among fatty foods such as oils, and wheatgerm (so wholemeal products contain more than low-extraction flour and bread). The US National Research Council recommend a daily intake of 30 International Units, which could be obtained from about 10g ($\frac{1}{3}$oz) of wheatgerm oil.

The vitamin is fairly stable to cooking, but up to 70 per cent may be destroyed by deep frying.

Vitamin F (see Essential Fatty Acids).

Vitamin K or **menaquinone** is essential for making the blood clot when you injure yourself. It can be produced by the natural bacteria in the intestine, so it is difficult to say how much is needed from food sources. However, green vegetables (kale, spinach, cauliflower, etc.) are all good sources.

Select Bibliography

This list is intended for those readers who would like to explore further any of the topics in this book. It is not in any way complete—a thorough bibliography of dietary systems would form a book in itself—but I think that all the titles represent a substantial amount of information. Classical and well known literary works have not been assigned to any particular edition, unless these are rather rare.

Classical
Apicius, M. Gavius. *De Re Coquinaria*, ed. Schuch, 1874
Balsdon, J. P. V. D. *Life and Leisure in Ancient Rome*, Bodley Head, London, 1969
Galen. *De Alimentorum Facultatibus*
Lucian of Samosata. *Satires* ('The Sale of Lives')
Ovid (P. Ovidius Naso). *Metamorphoses*, book 15
Petronius (G. Petronius Arbiter). *Satyricon* (particularly 'Trimalchio's Feast')
Plato. *Phaedo*
Seneca, Lucius Annaeus. *Letters*, no 108

History
Anon. *In this Tretyse that is Cleped Governayle of Helthe*, 1489. Facsimile ed. Da Capo Press, New York, 1969
Arbuthnot, Dr John. *Essay Concerning the Nature of Ailments*, London, 1731
Boord (Borde), Andrew. *The Breviarie of Health*, 1557
Brushfield, T. N. *The Salmon Clause in the Indentures of Apprentices* J. Historic. Soc. of Chester 1897, VI part 1

Burritt, Elihu. *A Walk from London to John O'Groats*, 1864
Burton, Robert. *The Anatomy of Melancholy*, 1621
Cornaro, Luigi. *Discorsi delle Vita Sobria* (about 1564) ed. Venice, 1620
Culpeper, Nicholas. *Complete Herbal*, 1654
Drummond, Sir Jack, and Wilbraham, Anne. *The Englishman's Food*, Jonathan Cape, London, 1957
Eden, Sir Frederick. *The State of the Poor*, 1797
Elyot, Sir Thomas. *The Castel of Helth*, 1539
Hanway, Jonas. *Letters on the Importance of the Rising Generation*, 1767
Harington, Sir John. *The Englishman's Doctor*, 1608
Hart, Dr James. *Klinike, or the Diet of the Diseased*, London, 1633
Hentzner, Paul. *A Journey into England* (1598), trans. Horace Walpole, 1757
Lemery, Louis. *A Treatise of Foodes in General*, London, 1706
Muffet (Moufet), Dr Thomas. *Health's Improvement*, London, 1655
Platt (Pratt), Sir Hugh. *Sundrie New and Artificial Remedies Against Famine*, 1596
Polwhele, Rev R. *History of Cornwall*, 1806
Pyke, Dr Magnus. *Townsman's Food*, Turnstile Press, London, 1952
Renner, H. D. *The Origin of Food Habits*, Faber, London, 1944
Simmonds, Peter L. *The Curiosities of Food*, Richard Bentley, London, 1859
Simoons, F. J. *Eat Not This Flesh*, University of Wisconsin, 1961
Slare, Frederick. *A Vindication of Sugars*, etc., 1715
Waleys, Thomas. *Moralitates*, 1330
Woodforde, Rev James. *The Diary of a Country Parson*, 1781
Young, Arthur. *The Farmer's Tour Through the East of England*, 1771

Vegetarianism
Anon. *On the Conduct of Man to Inferior Animals*, Manchester, 1797

Axon, William E. A. *Vegetarianism and the Intellectual Life*, Vegetarian Society, 1894

Barkas, Janet. *The Vegetable Passion*, Routledge & Kegan Paul, London, 1975

Besant, Annie. *Vegetarianism in the Light of Theosophy*, 1932

Broadbent, Albert (ed.). *The Vegetarian Textbook*, Vegetarian Society, Manchester, 1903

Crosby, Ernest, and Reclus, Elisée. *The Meat Fetish*, London, 1905

Densmore, Dr Emmet. *The Natural Food of Man*, London, 1890; *How Nature Cures*, 1892; *Fruit as Food*, 1892; *The Food of Paradise*, 1892

'Domestica'. *The Vegetist's Dietary*, 1884

Forward, Charles W. *The Vegetarian Birthday Book*, Ideal Publishing Union, London, 1898

Graham, Sylvester. *Lectures in the Science of Human Life*, 1839

Kingsford, Anna. *The Perfect Way in Diet*, London, 1881

Metcalfe, Rev William. *Abstinence from the Flesh of Animals*, 1821

Nawell, F. D. *Colds—Their Cause and Natural Cure*, Manchester, 1903

Newman, Francis W. *Vegetarianism*, Frasers Magazine, February 1875

Newton, John F. *The Return to Nature*, 1811

Oldfield, Dr Josiah. *Eat and Be Happy*, Methuen, London, 1929

Rosenberg, Theodor. *Fleisch oder Pflanzenkost*, Erlangen, 1900

Shelley, Percy B. *A Vindication of Natural Diet*, 1813; *Essay on the Vegetable Diet*, 1814: *Queen Mab* (1813) book 8

Tolstoy, Count Leo. *The First Step*. Trans. Aylmer Maude, Manchester, 1900

'Vegetaria'. *Medical and Scientific Testimony in Favour of a Vegetarian Diet* (undated, about 1900)

'Vegetarian'. *Stomach-Worship*, 1881

Werner, Heinrich. *Der Vegetärismus in Gegensatze zur Modernen Ernährungstheorie*, Erlangen, 1899

Other Systems

Anon. *The Biochemic Handbook*, New Era Laboratories, London, 1969

Atkins, Dr R. C. *Dr Atkins' Diet Revolution*, David McKay, 1972

Bell, Dr Robert. *Cancer: Its Cause and Treatment Without Operation*, London, 1903; *Dietetics and Hygienics Versus Disease*, Psychotherapeutic Society, London, 1910

Bieler, Dr Henry G. *Food Is Your Best Medicine*, Neville Spearman, London, 1968

Bircher-Benner, Maximilian. *The Prevention of Incurable Disease*, J. Clarke, London, 1959

Brandt, Joanna. *The Grape Cure*, Provoker Press, Ontario, 1930

Carter, Richard. *Your Food and Your Health*, Harper & Row, New York, 1964

Dewey, Dr Edward H. *The No-Breakfast Plan and the Fasting Cure*, Meadville, Pa., 1900

Fletcher, Horace. *The New Glutton or Epicure*, 1903; *The A.B.-Z. of our Own Nutrition*, 1903; *Fletcherism: What It Is; or How I Became Young at Sixty*, 1913

Glass, Justine. *Eat and Stay Young*, Peter Owens, London, 1956

Hay, Dr William H. *Health Via Food*, Harrap, London, 1934

Jarvis, De Forest C. *Folk Medicine*, W. H. Allen, London, 1960

Kordel, Lelord. *Eat Your Troubles Away*, Herbert Jenkins, London, 1956

Mellor, Constance. *Natural Remedies for Common Ailments*, C. W. Daniel, London, 1973

Oakley, E. Gilbert. *Better Health from Health Foods and Herbs*, Max Parrish, London, 1962

Sams, Craig. *About Macrobiotics*, Thorson, London, 1972

Sandlands, J. P. *Health—a Royal Road to It*, Felling-on-Tyne, 1909

Scott, Cyril. *Victory Over Cancer, Without Radium or Surgery*, Health Science Press, Rustington, 1969

Shelton, Herbert M. *Superior Nutrition*, Dr Shelton's Health School, Texas, 1951

Meat-eating

Kitchiner, Dr William. *The Art of Invigorating and Prolonging Life, etc.*, 1821; *Peptic Precepts* and *The Cook's Oracle*, 1821

Moncriff, Bernard. *The Philosophy of the Stomach*, London, 1856

Parry, Dr Thomas. *On Diet, With Its Influence on Man*, Highley, London, 1844

Stuart, Elma. *What Must I Do to Get Well?* (undated)

General Nutrition

American Medical Association. *Handbook of Nutrition*, 2nd. ed., H. K. Lewis, London, 1951

Bender, Dr Arnold E. *A Dictionary of Nutrition and Food Technology*, 3rd ed., Butterworths, London, 1968; *Nutrition and Dietetic Foods*, Leonard Hill, London, 1973

Blyth, Alexander W. *Diet in Relation to Health and Work*, William Clowes, London, 1884

Bogert, L. J., Briggs, G. M., and Calloway, D. H. *Nutrition and Physical Fitness*, W. B. Saunders, Philadelphia, 9th ed. 1973

Cullen, Dr William. *First Lines in the Practice of Physic*, Edinburgh, 1786

Cuvier, Baron George. *Règne Animal Distribué d'après son Organisation*, 1817

Davidson, Passmore and Brock. *Human Nutrition and Dietetics*, Churchill Livingstone, 5th ed., 1973

Drummond, Sir Jack C. *Chemistry and Man* (section 4), E. & F. N. Spon, London, 1953

Funk, Casimir. *The Vitamines*, 1914

Hanway, Jonas. *An Essay on Tea*, 1757

Hyatt-Woolf, Charles. *Truths About Things We Live On and Daily Use*, London, 1910; *Food Frauds and Foods That Feed*, London, 1897

Liebig, Baron Justus. *Chemistry in its Application to Agriculture and Physiology*, London, 1840; *The Chemistry of Animals*, London, 1842; *Chemical Researches on Meat and its Preparation for Food*, London, 1847

McCance, R. A., and Widdowson, E. M. *The Composition of Foods*, HMSO (MRC Special Report 297), 1960

Mackarness, Dr Richard. *Not All In the Mind*, Pan Books, London, 1976

Marks, Dr John. *A Guide to the Vitamins*, Medical and Technical Publications, Lancaster, 1975

Metchnikoff, Ilya (Elie). *Etudes sur la Nature Humaine*, 1903. Trans. P. Chalmers Mitchell as *The Nature of Man*, Heinemann, London, 1903

Pyke, Dr Magnus. *Industrial Nutrition*, MacDonald & Evans, 1950

Rodale, J. I. *A Complete Guide to the Vitamins*, Rodale Press, Berkhamsted, 1968

Sinclair, Hugh M., and Hollingsworth, Dorothy F. *Hutchinson's Food and the Principles of Nutrition*, Edward Arnold, London, 12th ed. 1969

Thompson, Sir Henry. *Food and Feeding*, 6th ed., 1891

Truman, Dr Matthew. *Food and its Influence on Health and Disease*, John Murray, 1842

Additions to Select Bibliography

Balsdon, J. P. V. D. *Life and Leisure in Ancient Rome*, McGraw-Hill, New York, 1969

Barkas, Janet. *The Vegetable Passion*, Scribner, New York, 1975

Bender, Dr Arnold E. *A Dictionary of Nutrition and Food Technology*, Shoe String Press, Hamden, Conn, 1968

Jarvis, De Forest C. *Folk Medicine*, Holt, Rinehart and Winston, New York, 1958

Rodale, J. I. *A Complete Guide to the Vitamins*, Rodale Press, Emmaus, Pa, and Berkhamsted, 1968

Index